THE TOP TEN DISEASES
OF ALL TIME

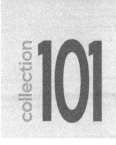

THE TOP TEN DISEASES OF ALL TIME

STACEY SMITH?

University of Ottawa Press
2023

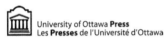

University of Ottawa **Press**
Les **Presses** de l'Université d'Ottawa

The University of Ottawa Press (UOP) is proud to be the oldest of the francophone university presses in Canada and the oldest bilingual university publisher in North America. Since 1936, UOP has been enriching intellectual and cultural discourse by producing peer-reviewed and award-winning books in the humanities and social sciences, in French and in English.

www.press.uOttawa.ca

Library and Archives Canada Cataloguing in Publication

Title: The top ten diseases of all time / Stacey Smith?.
Names: Smith?, Stacey, 1972 October 28- author.
Series: Collection 101 (Ottawa, Ont.)
Description: Series statement: Collection 101 | Includes bibliographical references and index.
Identifiers: Canadiana (print) 20230501567 | Canadiana (ebook) 20230501605 | ISBN 9780776640600
(softcover) | ISBN 9780776640617 (EPUB) | ISBN 9780776640624 (PDF)
Subjects: LCSH: Communicable diseases—History. | LCSH: Communicable diseases—Social aspects.
Classification: LCC RC111 .S65 2023 | DDC 616.909—dc23

Legal Deposit: Fourth Quarter 2023
Library and Archives Canada

Production Team

Copy editing   Céline Parent
Proofreading   Robbie McCaw
Typesetting   Nord Compo

The University of Ottawa Press gratefully acknowledges the support extended to its publishing list by the Government of Canada, the Canada Council for the Arts, the Ontario Arts Council, the Federation for the Humanities and Social Sciences through the Scholarly Book Awards and the Social Sciences and Humanities Research Council, and by the University of Ottawa.

  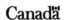

u Ottawa

*Dedicated to all the people who died from infectious diseases
and whose names have been lost to history*

Contents

List of Illustrations

List of Tables

Preface

When I first suggested this book, based on a workshop I'd been running since 2016,* the idea of pandemics was mostly a thought experiment or something confined to history and the nebulous *elsewhere*. I've been studying infectious diseases, vaccines, and pandemics for several decades (and even lived through a couple myself, such as getting caught in the 2014 African Ebola outbreak), but even I never expected a pandemic in my own backyard. With COVID-19 having affected every corner of the globe, concepts like a disease's reproduction number and herd immunity are no longer just the stuff of ivory-tower academics.

Every disease has its own quirks and eccentricities, but there are also broad patterns that many pandemics follow, making them quite predictable in some ways—and entirely unpredictable in others. But knowing when we might be in one situation versus the other is critical, and often we can do very well at predicting a lot, based on a little. I'm a professor of biomathematics by training, but many of you will be pleased to hear that there is no mathematics in this book. Instead, this is a story about patterns and history, about the way disease reshapes societies and cultures, about death and innovation. (So a lot less scary than it could be, for all the math-phobes out there.)

Part of the reason for this book's existence, aside from the fascination that I and many others have with disease as a force of nature and an agent of change, is that I had never been able to track down the numbers for the top ten diseases of all time. There are Buzzfeed lists and so forth, but none had reliable numbers, no two lists ever seemed to agree with each other, and they never included their sources. Here, I've attempted to find sources for all the numbers—with the caveats that a) some of the numbers are by necessity estimates, which are the only available options when dealing with epidemics throughout history, and b) some are broad ranges, although fortunately those ranges don't really overlap. These may not be perfect, but they're better than anything we've had thus far. At the very least, I've shown my work, so you can judge for yourself.

This book is more than just the numbers, however. Humans are fascinating creatures, especially when they're afraid. Diseases ramp up that fear, forcing us into corners we might not always choose if we were more rational. That's

---

* If you google, you can find a YouTube video of me giving the workshop that evolved into this book...in January 2020. That's right, weeks before COVID hit, I was warning about the ability of pandemics to reshape societies. It was a different time, so you'll find me under a different name and different gender.

pretty clear from the experiences during COVID-19, as the epidemic pokes at all our weaknesses, but this turns out to have been just as true over the entirety of human history. Along the way, there are also moments of greatness and wonder, as those corners we're forced into can sometimes produce amazing responses and lead to unexpected world-changing outcomes.

One of the big fears around disease is just how random it is. You can be going about your business, not doing anything wrong, and simply be cut down. This is a supremely uncomfortable feeling for most humans, so we expend a lot of energy attempting to impose control—or at least the illusion of control—over infectious diseases and our role in them. A great many religious practices evolved to combat diseases: pork was *verboten* in many religions for the very sensible reason that pigs carried diseases, so the message needed to be spread that pigs should not be eaten.[1] Religion is a very good way to both disseminate and inculcate a message to a vast number of people, including distant descendants.[2] Our funeral practices—burying bodies six feet underground—are the result of the bubonic plague, because six feet was determined to be the depth at which the virus could no longer be transmitted from a dead body.[3] Monogamy was a great way of avoiding sexually transmitted diseases in a time before antibiotics or laboratory testing. Today's conspiracy theories are a comforting way to impose a form of control on an unpredictable world. "Hey, maybe the government is out to get me, but at least that means someone has their hand on the rudder, which is a lot better than the alternative of no one being in charge in a chaotic and random world!" This thought process allows us to "reason" our way out of feeling at risk.

Diseases have been a driver of so many of our cultural practices that we often forget their origins and continue the practices long after the need for them has faded. But sometimes the reverse happens: we stop doing the things that keep us safe because the disease has seemingly disappeared, only to create an opening for it to come roaring back.

Background

Infectious diseases have been a part of the human condition since time immemorial. Some, such as mumps or chickenpox, usually have mild symptoms and mostly lead to recovery. Others, such as HIV, tuberculosis, or malaria, are responsible for millions of deaths each year. The 1918 Spanish influenza pandemic killed millions of people in the space of six months.[4]

Sociological upheavals following the Black Death led to the demise of the church as an all-powerful institution,[5] the destruction of the serf system, and the subsequent creation of labour movements and colonialism.[6] The universal symbol for a medic—the Rod of Asclepius—is an image of worms wrapped around a stick, because that was the only way to remove Guinea worms from the body, so having a stick meant you were a doctor.[7] Malaria was one of four diseases that were targeted for eradication in the twentieth century;[8] the failure to do so arose directly from the conception of the environmental movement.[9]

Despite its massive death toll, smallpox remains the only successfully eradicated human disease (but not for long!), thanks to a successful vaccine, photographic-recognition cards, and forced vaccinations of whole villages in

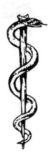

Figure 0.1. The Rod of Asclepius.
Source: Public domain.

the former Yugoslavia.[10] Other momentous achievements are the virtual disappearance of erstwhile disabling and lethal diseases such as diphtheria, tetanus, paralytic poliomyelitis, pertussis, measles, mumps, rubella, and invasive *H. influenzae b*.[11] While these victories are an undeniable positive, they bring up issues of individual rights versus public good that remain relevant today.

Throughout the ages, infectious diseases have been the source of fear and superstition. They continue to pose a threat, from the irritation of the cold and flu season to the potential extinction of our species. But what are the worst of the worst? In order to understand what that means, we need a measure of what constitutes "bad." A disease that doesn't kill but leaves you disfigured and unable to work (as elephantiasis does) inflicts enormous suffering, both personally and economically. Those things are hugely important, but they're not the focus of this book.

Here, we will centre on the biggest, baddest diseases of all time using the sheer number of deaths as the measure of damage. Largely, that's because this is an easily definable metric, although it ignores the relative population sizes. The Mexican haemorrhagic fevers of the sixteenth century might have reduced the population by 28 million, a lot fewer than Spanish influenza's 50–100 million deaths—except that the Mexican population was only 30 million when it started,[12] making for a devastating 93% death toll, whereas the twentieth century's largest pandemic "only" killed 5.5% of the world's population; this would be equivalent to 350 million deaths today.

Nevertheless, this metric is the hill we're going to die on, possibly very quickly and quite painfully. However, by its very nature, focusing on the sheer number of deaths ignores a large number of diseases, either because they fall just outside the top ten or because their primary symptoms do not involve death. It's worth mentioning a few of these before we go on.

Some of the Diseases that Don't Fall into the Top Ten

The tale of diseases and their effects on society is by turns complex and overarching and has a surprising number of recognizable names attached.

For example, syphilis was known as the musician's disease, because a goodly chunk of composers, particularly in the late eighteenth and early nineteenth century, are thought to have died from it, including Smetana, Wolf, Joplin, Delius,[13] Donizetti,[14] Schubert, Schumann, and others.[15]

Historical attempts to fight infectious diseases, both successful and not, are equally fascinating. In the case of syphilis, early treatment was with mercury, which was unpleasant and often toxic, leading to neuropathies, kidney failure, loss of teeth, and eventual death by mercury poisoning.[16] Syphilis was finally slowed in the mid-twentieth century by the advent of penicillin.[17] Penicillin was one of those happy accidents of science, discovered in 1928 when Alexander Fleming—who was often described as a careless lab technician—returned from a two-week vacation to find that a mould had grown on an accidentally contaminated staphylococcus culture plate, and the culture had prevented the growth of the staphylococci.[18] Penicillin's role in reducing the incidence of diseases like syphilis was responsible for the sexual revolution of the 1960s, even more than the birth control pill.[19]

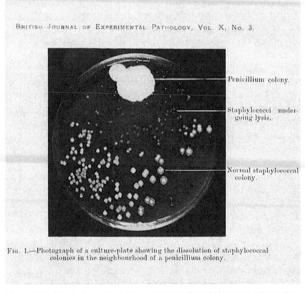

Figure 0.2. Fleming's accidentally contaminated staphylococcus culture plate.
Source: A. Fleming, "On the Antibacterial Action of Cultures of a Penicillium, with Special Reference to Their Use in the Isolation of *B. influenzae*," *British Journal of Experimental Pathology* 10, no. 3 (1929): 226–236.

You might have heard of a group of diseases called the Neglected Tropical Diseases (NTDs). This isn't just a generic title for all the forgotten diseases in the world; it's a specific designation on behalf of the World Health Organization for 21 particular diseases that qualify for neglected status.[20] Collectively, these diseases infect about one sixth of the world's population.

Table 0.1. The neglected tropical diseases

Infection		Global prevalence (millions)	Population at risk
Soil-transmitted helminths (aka "the unholy trinity")	Hookworm	807	5.1 billion
	Roundworm	604	3.2 billion
	Whipworm	576	3.2 billion
Foodborne trematodiases (*worms found in meat*)		56	750 million
Tapeworms	Taeniasis	50	N/A
	Cysticercosis	40	N/A
	Echinococcosis	1	6 billion
Dengue		528	2.5 billion
Schistosomiasis		207	779 million
Elephantitis		120	1.3 billion
Trachoma		84	590 million
River blindness		37	90 million
Leishmaniasis		12	350 million
Chagas disease		8–9	25 million
Yaws		2.5	434 million
Chikungunya		2	793 million
Leprosy		0.4	N/A
Sleeping sickness		0.3	60 million
Rabies		0.06	3 billion
Guinea-worm disease		0.0001	N/A
Buruli ulcer		N/A	N/A

Source: S.M. Bartsch et al., "The Global Economic and Health Burden of Human Hookworm Infection," *PLoS Neglected Tropical Diseases* 10 (2016): e0004922; A.D. Kealey and R.J. Smith?, "Neglected Tropical Diseases: Infection, Modeling, and Control," *Journal of Health Care for the Poor and Underserved* 21 (2010): 53–69.

Approximately 5.1 billion people—more than half the population of Earth—are at risk for hookworm alone, of which half a billion are currently infected.[21] What characterizes these particular diseases is that—unlike more sensational diseases like HIV/AIDS, measles, and TB that we'll be talking about—they don't kill huge numbers of people (collectively, the NTDs kill about 200,000 people per year,[22] although that's still not nothing). Instead, they're responsible for massive levels of disfigurement and disability, impairing childhood development and economic productivity. They're found in every tropical country (including Australia) and yet are neglected at the community, national, and international levels, largely because they affect the poor, the powerless, and the stigmatized.[23]

For example, Chagas disease kills 50,000 people a year (far more than West Nile virus, bird flu, and swine flu combined), but you probably haven't heard of it because it's a disease of the poor. If your house is made of sticks, the bugs that carry the disease burrow through your walls and bite you under the eye. But if you can afford plaster for your walls, then you're safe. So it's a widespread disease in poor rural South America (where the average lifespan of a dog is about two years, thanks to the disease), but it doesn't kill anyone who might be in a position to lobby governments, advocate for medical interventions, or mobilize advertising campaigns.[24]

Rather than simply count deaths, the World Health Organization has developed a measure of the number of years of life lost from premature death or disability, or DALYs (Disability-Adjusted Life Years). This can also be used to measure the cost-effectiveness of interventions.[25] The number of DALYs per year for HIV/AIDS is 40.1 million. That is, without HIV/AIDS we'd have about 40,100,000 years of healthy life back. Malaria's DALY was 33.4 million in 2019, and TB's was 66 million. Although generally non-fatal, diarrhoeal diseases accounted for a whopping 79 million DALYs. But NTDs also have a significant burden on the world, with collective DALYs of 14.9 million.[26] So despite being neglected, the NTDs are still an enormous problem for a great many people.

Treatments exist for some NTDs, although in practice control often occurs using far less "sexy" methods, such as mass deworming in schools, insecticides, safe water, and, in some cases, arsenic and amputation. (Seriously: arsenic is still used to treat sleeping sickness, while the only treatment for the Buruli ulcer is to amputate infected limbs. NTDs ain't pretty.) Part of the problem is that there is no money in them: why would a profit-driven pharmaceutical company waste time developing treatments for diseases whose sufferers can't pay?

Fortunately, there are a couple of success stories. Guinea-worm disease has been all but eliminated, despite having no vaccine, no drug, and no immunity.* Instead, behaviour changes (convincing people not to put infected limbs in the water, distributing cloth filters to villages, and outfitting nomadic people with drinking pipes) have led to a massive reduction in cases—from 3.5 million in 1989 to just 13 in 2022—and already eliminated the disease from Asia and the Middle East.[27] How did this miraculous feat get accomplished? It's thanks to the efforts of one man: former U.S. president Jimmy Carter, who did the unglamorous but important work of mobilizing public–private partnerships, delivering education messages to remote populations, and even negotiating a "Guinea-worm ceasefire" in the Sudan civil war so that NGOs could go in and educate those most at risk. As a result, Guinea-worm disease has been almost eradicated from the planet. It is not only going to be the first parasitic disease to be eradicated, it is also going to be the first to be eliminated using behaviour changes alone. That's an incredible achievement.

Another success story is river blindness. In 1974, the West African river blindness program was developed as a collaboration between the

---

* A vaccine is usually given in advance in order to prevent infection. Drugs are usually given after infection, to treat the disease or its symptoms. Immunity is a property of the body and comes in two forms: innate (we're immune to some diseases at birth, thanks to genetics) and adaptive (the immune system can learn from previous infections and design defences against them for future protection).

World Health Organization, the World Bank, the United Nations, and 20 donor countries and agencies. Mathematical modelling was used at the outset to predict long-term outcomes; by including modelling in the design of the program, sceptical donors were convinced that control was feasible. When the anti-parasite drug ivermectin was made available in the late eighties, partway through the program, mathematical models were able to adapt to its inclusion. The program was completed in 2002, with 40 million people treated, blindness prevented in 600,000 people, and 25 million hectares of land made safe for resettlement.[28]

The Academic Part of This Book

We've played a little loose with the definitions of what counts as a "disease," as the same infection can be counted twice. However, we take the view that the cultural understanding of a disease is just as important as the science, so our view is that if the outbreaks had distinct names and were separated in history, then they're distinct epidemics. Chapters 5 and 7 are both about plague, but almost a thousand years separates the two. Had the 2009 swine flu epidemic had a greater death toll, we'd be considering that as separate from the 1918 pandemic influenza, despite both being H1N1 flu. Conversely, while measles has been around for centuries, it's understood as a single entity, and we've treated it as such.

While infectious diseases are simultaneously terrifying and captivating, one of the features of this book is to nail down the numbers. No other single source has done this; a number of websites claim to, but their numbers are contradictory and are not supported by research. The aim of this work is to provide a level of scientific rigour unavailable in other outlets. Along the way, we'll discover fun facts about the influence of particular diseases on societies both distant and modern, as well as learn about the worst thing the human race has ever encountered. Hint: it's not zombies...

A Word about COVID-19

At the time of writing, deaths from COVID-19 have just passed *6.95 million*. You might notice that this isn't even close to qualifying it for the #10 disease in this list. The impact of COVID-19 on changing our society has not been fully played out yet, so it will have to be left to future authors to determine its structural effects on our culture. However, we'll contrast some of the impacts of other diseases against our current COVID epidemic, so in many ways COVID-19 has been woven into the fabric of a lot of this book.

Acknowledgements

This book would have been a lot poorer without Laura Bruce, who made a fantastic research assistant, or Gabriel(le) DeRooy, whose proofread turned the final draft into the penultimate one. My thanks, as always, to Anthony Wilson for his structural insights. I'm incredibly grateful to

Mark Nelson and David Fisman, whose comments and insights were magnificent, forcing me to work hard to justify a lot of things and also giving me some fascinating new directions. I can't thank them enough for holding my feet to the fire. Enormous thanks to the University of Ottawa Press team—Lara Mainville, Caroline Boudreau, Laurence Sylvain, Benoit Deneault—for being willing to go with the idea in the first place and shepherding it through. Thanks to Laura, Mélan, Red, Torben, and Rav for moral support. And a final word of thanks to the many people (friends, family, and strangers in my hair salon) for whom "Guess the top ten diseases of all time!" became the best pub quiz we'd ever played and whose questions helped me shape and reshape this book.

Notes

1. H.R. Gamble, "Parasites Associated with Pork and Pork Products," *Revue scientifique et technique-Office international des épizooties* 16, no.2 (1997): 496–506.
2. K. Orman, *The Black Archive: Pyramids of Mars* (Edinburgh: Obverse Books, 2017).
3. D. Defoe, *A Journal of the Plague Year* (London: E. Nutt, 1722).
4. N.P. Johnson and J. Mueller, "Updating the Accounts: Global Mortality of the 1918–1920 'Spanish' Influenza Pandemic," *Bulletin of the History of Medicine* 76 (2002): 105–115.
5. W.J. Dohar, *The Black Death and Pastoral Leadership* (Philadelphia: University of Pennsylvania Press, 2018).
6. E.D. Domar, "The Causes of Slavery or Serfdom: A Hypothesis," *Journal of Economic History* 30, no. 1 (1970): 18–32.
7. R.J. Smith? et al., "A Mathematical Model for the Eradication of Guinea Worm Disease," in *Understanding the Dynamics of Emerging and Re-Emerging Infectious Diseases Using Mathematical Models*, ed. S. Mushayabasa and C. Bhunu (Kerala: Transworld Research, 2012), 133–162.
8. R. Smith?, "Did We Eradicate SARS? Lessons Learned and the Way Forward," *American Journal of Biomedical Science and Research* 6, no. 2 (2019): 152–155.
9. M. Finkel, "Stopping a Global Killer," *National Geographic*, 6 June 2007.
10. F. Fenner et al., *Smallpox and Its Eradication* (Geneva: World Health Organization, 1988).
11. F.E. André, "Vaccinology: Past Achievements, Present Roadblocks and Future Promises," *Vaccine* 21, no. 7–8 (2003): 593–595.
12. S.F. Cook and L.B. Simpson, "The Population of Central Mexico in the Sixteenth Century," *Ibero Americana* 31 (1948):43–55.
13. M.K. Pedro, F.M. Germiniani, and H.A. Teive, "Neurosyphilis and Classical Music: The Great Composers and 'The Great Imitator,'" *Arquivos de neuro-psiquiatria* 76 (2018): 791–794.
14. E. Peschel and R. Peschel, "R. Donizetti and the music of mental derangement: Anna Bolena, Lucia di Lammermoor, and the composer's neurobiological illness," *The Yale Journal of Biology and Medicine* 65, no. 3 (1992): 189.
15. C. Franzen, "Syphilis in Composers and Musicians—Mozart, Beethoven, Paganini, Schubert, Schumann, Smetana," *European Journal of Clinical Microbiology & Infectious Diseases* 27, no. 12 (2008): 1151–1157.
16. J. Frith, "Syphilis—Its Early History and Treatment until Penicillin and the Debate on Its Origins," *Journal of Military and Veterans' Health* 20 (2012): 49–58.
17. J. Frith, "Syphilis—Its Early History and Treatment until Penicillin and the Debate on Its Origins".
18. K. Kalvaitis, "Penicillin: An Accidental Discovery Changed the Course of Medicine," *Endocrine Today* (10 August 2008).

19. S. Ferro, "Did Penicillin Kickstart the Sexual Revolution?," *Popular Science* (28 January 2013).

20. P.J. Hotez et al., "The Neglected Tropical Diseases: The Ancient Afflictions of Stigma and Poverty and the Prospects for Their control and Elimination," in *Hot Topics in Infection and Immunity in Children III*, ed. A.J. Pollard and A. Finn (New York: Springer, 2006), 23–33.

21. S.M. Bartsch et al., "The Global Economic and Health Burden of Human Hookworm Infection," *PLoS Neglected Tropical Diseases* 10 (2016): e0004922.

22. D.A. Álvarez-Hernández et al., "Overcoming the Global Burden of Neglected Tropical Diseases," *Therapeutic Advances in Infectious Disease* 7 (2020): 1–3.

23. M.G. Weiss, "Stigma and the Social Burden of Neglected Tropical Diseases," *PLoS Neglected Tropical Diseases* 2, no. 5 (2008): e237.

24. R. Smith?, "Neglected Tropical Diseases—How Mathematics Can Help," in *Mathematics of Planet Earth: Mathematicians Reflect on How to Discover, Organize, and Protect Our Planet*, ed. H.G. Kaper and C. Rousseau (Philadelphia: Society for Industrial and Applied Mathematics, 2015), 183–184.

25. F. Sassi, "Calculating QALYs, Comparing QALY and DALY Calculations," *Health Policy and Planning* 21, no. 5 (2006): 402–408.

26. Global Health Estimates: Leading Causes of DALYs, Disease Burden, 2000–2019, *World Health Organization*, https://www.who.int/data/gho/data/themes/mortality-and-global-health-estimates/global-health-estimates-leading-causes-of-dalys.

27. S.A. Guagliardo et al., "Surveillance of Human Guinea Worm in Chad, 2010–2018," *The American Journal of Tropical Medicine and Hygiene* 105, no. 1 (2021): 188.

28. M.G. Basáñez et al., "River Blindness: A Success Story under Threat?," *PLoS Medicine* 3, no. 9 (2006): e371.

10 **The Third Plague**

I t started in a province in China, but it wasn't contained there for long. Spreading outward, the disease first hit neighbouring countries, before travelling further and faster than any such disease had ever managed, thanks to technological developments in travel previously unseen in any pandemic. Before long, the disease had crossed continents, eventually making its way to almost every corner of the planet, killing millions in its wake. But that's enough about COVID-19, let's talk about the Third Plague.

As the name suggests, there have been three major plague epidemics throughout history. The first was the Justinianic Plague of Roman times (see chapter 7), while the second was the Black Death of the Middle Ages (see chapter 5). As mentioned in the introduction, despite having the same underlying bacteria, we're considering these to be distinct epidemics because they are separated in time and culture, they have distinct names, and—due to differing virulence, symptoms, and reasoning about the distances that rats can travel—they might possibly be different diseases.[1]

The Third Plague originated in 1855 after a mining boom resulted in a rapid influx of workers in Yunnan Province, China, to mine copper and other minerals, due to rising demand in the second half of the nineteenth century. From Yunnan in the Southwest, it was brought to coastal regions due to the growing opium trade, which began after 1840.[2] From the coasts of China, then-new steamship navigation moved humans around at unprecedented rates, taking rats and the disease with them.[3] However, it was not known at the time that rats were the cause of the disease, other than their bodies being a "warning sign" that it was present; the thinking was that the disease was caused by miasmas: noxious poisons emanating from the soil or bodies of plague victims.[4] The case-fatality rate—a measure of how likely you are to die if you actually catch the disease[5]—was greater than 93%.[6]

Plague is spread by fleas, which acquire the bacteria (known as *Yersinia pestis*) by sucking blood from an infected rodent. Bacteria quickly multiply and block the alimentary canal in the gut of the fleas. The fleas transmit the bacteria to new rodent hosts by regurgitating clotted blood.[7] Symptoms include fever, chills, headache, body pains, weakness, vomiting, and nausea, followed by painful swollen lymph nodes. The bubonic form—so named for the buboes, or pustules, that form on the skin of the infected[8]—is the most common and is fatal in 50%–90% of cases, which is incredibly high.

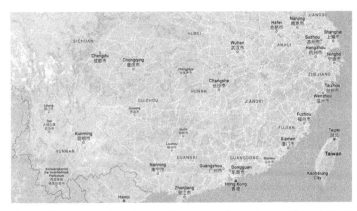

Figure 10.1. Map of southern China and its provinces (Guangzhou and Guangdong are in the South, while Yunnan is in the West).

Source: Google Maps.

There are two other types of plague: pneumonic plague, which has a mortality rate of 90%–95%, and septicemic plague, with a mortality rate near 100%.[9] Pneumonic plague is characterized by a fulminating onset of symptoms—the body becomes overwhelmed by attack—and is rapidly fatal when left untreated.[10] Indeed, so fast were some infections that people who went to bed healthy would be dead by morning.[11] Pneumonic plague leads to inter-human transmission, as opposed to just infection by rats, but the high virulence means the disease usually burns itself out.[12]

The disease spread from Guangdong Province in China to nearby Hong Kong due to the unrestricted movement of workers and boats arriving in Hong Kong.[13] This coincided with the replacement of junks with steam-ships, making travel between infected ports faster and more convenient.[14] On March 2, 1894, a Chinese procession was held in Hong Kong, which involved the arrival of 40,000 labourers from Canton.[15] Around the same time, Chinese workers who had been away celebrating the Qingming Festival returned from Guangzhou to Hong Kong in large numbers.[16] A dry spell in the summer of 1894 meant that much of the filth had not been washed away by the rains. This led to an increase in the number of rats in the streets, creating conditions for an outbreak.[17]

The Hong Kong government asked Dr. Alexander Rennie, the consular surgeon for Canton, to identify whether the new disease really was the bubonic plague. Rennie identified it but said that it would not be partic-ularly contagious except to those living in conditions involving filth, poor ventilation, or poor water supply.[18] Unfortunately, this turned out to be quite a number of people.

Attempts by the British to control the disease did not go well. For a time, the British in Hong Kong placed plague patients on boats because it was believed that people living and working on the water were not exposed to the miasma that rose from the ground.[19] The Chinese would hide their sick from the authorities, and infected bodies would be thrown out at night to avoid detection.[20] Patients were also cooled with ice, but many Chinese thought that such extreme cold would only exaggerate the infection, so they fled Hong Kong, taking the disease with them.[21] Chinese ladies were reluctant to let foreign doctors into their boudoir,[22] while rumours of white soldiers wishing to rape Chinese women abounded.[23] Tensions grew so high that doctors had to carry pistols to protect themselves.[24]

Britain was the world's dominant maritime and imperial power of the day, making it the inadvertent engine helping to move plague around the world. Most of the cases and deaths occurred within the British Empire, with British ships calling at international ports the unwitting instruments in the rapid dissemination of *Y. pestis*.[25] Europe was hit less hard, as rats were not generally found outside of warehouses in ports and in a few towns.[26] The Third Plague had significant effects on societies it touched, both positive and negative, contributing directly to anti-Asian prejudice in the United States, the creation of apartheid in South Africa, and the growth of public-health services in Brazil.[27]

Plague travelled from Hong Kong to British-occupied Bombay in 1896,[28] where the story was quite similar. Tradesmen who worked near grain silos were at risk from exposure to rats, but the bigger risk was to the urban poor, who were living in overcrowded conditions.[29] The disease, the authorities maintained, would soon be stamped out. However, initially the British had little idea of how to tackle the epidemic,[30] and the population resisted their attempts to do so. Indians saw hospitals and doctors as agents of the plague, desiring to either kill or infect them on Crown orders.[31]

A deputation—including Mehdi Hasan Khan, from the old Avadh royal family—met with Sir Antony MacDonnell, the lieutenant-governor of the Northwestern provinces. They told MacDonnell that they "considered the plague a far less evil than separation from plague-stricken members of their families; that plague was a God-sent dispensation, against which they were not at all sure it was not impious to contend; and that happen what might, they would never permit the segregation of their women or the administration of European drugs to their families."[32]

It was eventually learned that cleaning and disinfecting was an essential part of plague control. Plague outbreaks could be contained or avoided in places in Bombay where it was possible to clean dwellings, houses, and streets.[33] However, these measures brought their own problems, as attempts to contain and treat the plague led to considerable backlash, including the assassination of the plague commissioner in 1897.[34]

Anti-European riots broke out on March 9, 1898. Plague huts were set on fire, and a hospital was almost razed to the ground after attempts to examine a 12-year-old Muslim girl.[35] When British troops were called in to help local medical officers, Indian resistance grew more creative. They memorized the inspection troops' routes to avoid being caught unaware and hid infected family members within chests and under clothing.[36]

India faced the most substantial casualties, and the epidemic was used as an excuse for repressive policies that sparked some revolt against the British.[37] A staggering *12.5 million* people died from the plague in India between 1898 and 1918.[38] This was five sixths of the global total, which has been estimated to be as high as *15 million*.[39] The extreme casualty list was in part because the advent of irrigation in previously dry areas (such as the Punjab) allowed plague to flourish.[40] Enormous death tolls caused some coastal villages to lose over a quarter of their population within two to three months.[41]

The situation in Africa saw similar problems, but with radically different approaches to disease management. European medical officers in Egypt were obliged to concede to local Islamic practice in their plague-control operations. Because Islamic law allowed only women to examine female corpses, officials trained Egyptian midwives and health assistants—known as *hakimas*—to identify plague symptoms and hired European women as midwives and physicians. The general civility with which plague-control operations were conducted in Egypt made plague sufferers and the population at large more comfortable and more open to Western biomedical practices.[42]

Conversely, when cases broke out in Cape Town, Black Africans were rounded up and removed, which kept the plague in check.[43] This was the first racial segregation in South Africa, and it set the country on the path towards apartheid. White segregationists argued for the partition on the grounds of sanitary requirements.[44]

Such health-related discrimination was not restricted to countries under British colonial rule. In the New World, the outbreak in San Francisco in 1904–1908 was the first in the United States.[45] It was denied by federal health authorities, and a racially motivated quarantine prevented even physicians from crossing into Chinatown to identify and help the sick.[46] California Governor Henry Gage denied the existence of plague in San Francisco, fearing that it would damage the city and state economy. Supportive newspapers began an intense defamation campaign against quarantine officer Joseph Kinyoun.[47] In response, the federal treasury intervened, creating a commission which determined that plague was indeed present.[48] Chinatown was placed under a second quarantine, and orders were given for no East Asians to cross the quarantine line. All persons of Asian heritage in Chinatown were to be inoculated with the then-new Haffkine vaccine, which was known to have severe side effects.[49]

However, the Chinese community invoked the Fourteenth Amendment, feeling that they were not receiving equal protection under the law in their resistance to what was perceived as an experimental vaccine. Federal Judge William W. Morrow ruled in favour of the Chinese, because the state of California was unable to prove that Chinese Americans were more susceptible to the disease than Anglo Americans. This position set a precedent for greater limits placed on public-health authorities seeking to isolate infected populations,[50] but it also emboldened white supremacists, who equated the "yellow peril" with the black plague.[51]

Further south, Brazilian sanitarian Oswaldo Cruz had stemmed the 1902 yellow fever epidemic, thanks to an intensive insecticide program to wipe out mosquitoes, despite there being no proof at the time that the disease was carried by them. Cruz turned his strategy of fighting disease vectors to plague in 1903, with a hunt for rats in Rio de Janeiro. Employees of the public-health directorate were given the goal of turning up at least 150 rats a month, under threat of dismissal, and the government began to buy rats from anyone who killed them.[52] Efforts to import and coordinate an anti-plague serum from Europe led to the creation of multiple public-health institutes in Brazil.[53]

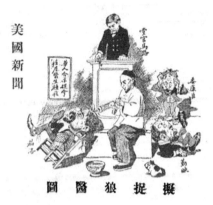

Figure 10.2. Political cartoon in a Chinese-language newspaper published in June 1900, depicting Joseph Kinyoun being injected in the head with the Haffkine vaccine. Nearby doctors are developing buboes from the inoculations.

Source: Present Status of Plague, with Historical Review, 1920.

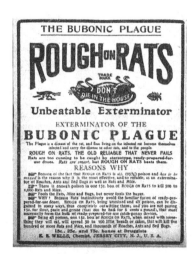

Figure 10.3. Newspaper ad for rat extermination to prevent plague.

Source: The New York Times, 14 April 1908.

Australia suffered no less than 12 outbreaks between 1900 and 1925.[54] By 1899, Nouméa in New Caledonia was declared a port of infection, with the disease arriving in Sydney in early 1900. However, the early warning gave authorities the chance to prepare. Dr. J. Ashburton Thompson—at the time the only trained epidemiologist in the entire country—undertook a two-pronged approach: as director of the board of health, he lobbied for government action, and he had his brother, a journalist at the *Daily Telegraph*, publish anonymously in the press.[55] Thompson was the first to show that the disease was spread by rats, bringing scientific scrutiny to public health.[56] Intensive cleaning and disinfecting programs were undertaken, with rats captured and poisoned in large numbers. Australia's example became instrumental in proving the importance of public-health departments and modern, sanitary, urban-planning principles.[57]

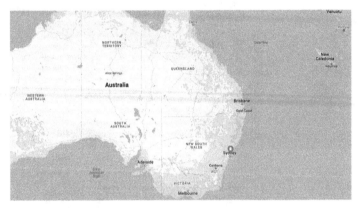

Figure 10.4. Map of Australia and New Caledonia.
Source: Google Maps.

The actual cause of the disease had not been understood for centuries, but the Third Plague coincided with a biomedical revolution: it was the era of vaccine development, novel discoveries, and identification of longstanding causes of diseases. However, it also pitted doctors against politicians. Doctors had the tools and obligations to help, but decision makers had to weigh medical risks against political and ideological imperatives.[58]

The strategy followed the three *i*'s: isolation, incineration, and inoculation, but each had their problems. As mentioned above, isolation (quarantine) engendered resentment—in part because the plague was largely not spread from human to human—encouraging people to hide the sick and the dead.[59] Incineration involved burning clothing, bedding, and sometimes entire dwellings of those suspected to be infected. This policy derived in part from older European public-health measures, specifically around smallpox, but it also created resentment among the poor, who had limited means. Additionally, it may have driven the rats away from areas where it was implemented, causing them to carry the plague elsewhere.[60] Incineration measures led to the great fire of 1900 in Honolulu, leaving 7,000 workers homeless.[61] Indeed, the Honolulu plague was a factor in Hawaii's status as a territory that eventually led to its statehood (unlike the Philippines);[62] in a confluence of two interconnected campaigns—one medical, one political—Hawaii gained territory status in Washington, DC, the very day the island's governor declared it free of the plague.[63]

Inoculation was the only one of the plague-control measures that could be attributed to the new science of immunology.[64] During the Hong Kong outbreak in 1894, Alexandre Yersin—who had been a student of Louis Pasteur, the father of microbiology and inventor of vaccines for rabies and anthrax—discovered the bacterium causing the plague, which bears his name (*Yersinia pestis*).[65] He was also able to show that the bacterial DNA was identical in rodents, suggesting a transmission route.[66] Japanese physician Shibasaburo Kitasato almost simultaneously identified *Y. pestis* as the pathogen* responsible for the plague, but his bacterial plates were unfortunately contaminated, which led to erroneous observations.[67] The two were initially credited as independent co-discoverers, but within a few years only Yersin was cited.[68]

In Bombay in 1897, French scientist Paul-Louis Simond and zoologist Waldemar Haffkine, a Ukrainian Jew in British employ, suggested that rats were a key vector.[69] In 1898, Simond put forward the theory that fleas could contain the plague bacillus.† In his experiment, Simond found that fleas transmitted plague among rats and, when hungry, to humans.[70] Skepticism surrounded Simond's findings, and the medical community largely ignored and dismissed his publication. If accepted, his work would have negated much of the anti-plague measures advocated by the medical community and enforced by the British Army. Although Ashburton Thompson subsequently showed that plague was spread by rats in Australia, it would be another eight years before Simond's work linking rats, fleas, and human infection gained acceptance and influenced proactive measures in India.[71]

Haffkine had previously developed a cholera vaccine, being the first vaccinologist to test a vaccine on himself in order to prove it was safe.[72] In 1897, he developed a practical and inexpensive anti-plague vaccine from a broth colony killed by heat[73] and again tested it on himself.[74] Volunteers at a local jail were used in a control test. All inoculated prisoners survived, while seven inmates in the control group died.[75] Unlike tetanus or diphtheria vaccines, which acted quickly, the Haffkine formulation had nasty side effects (as seen in the inhabitants of San Francisco's Chinatown, mentioned above) and did not provide complete protection, though it was said to have reduced risk by up to 50%.[76] Another major limit of Haffkine's vaccine was the lack of protection against pulmonary forms of plague.[77] However, he was proclaimed "the saviour of mankind"[78] by British surgeon Joseph Lister (the father of modern surgery).

The accidental contamination of a bottle of vaccines by an assistant caused the death of 19, leaving a lasting stain on Haffkine's legacy.[79] Sir Ronald Ross, who later developed insights into malaria, issued a stark warning when lobbying to overturn this injustice. In a moment of prescience, he said that misplaced fears of deadly vaccination threatened to undermine public trust in vaccines at a time when at least 50,000 people were dying every week from plague.[80]

---

* A pathogen is any organism causing disease in its host. These include bacteria, viruses, fungi, worms, protozoa, and prions.
† Bacillus are rod-shaped bacteria, which exhibit a wide range of physiological abilities, allowing them to live in every natural environment. There are 266 named species.

Haffkine had been revered in some parts of India, but as colonial health officials began to recommend the use of his vaccine, the public opposed its introduction.[81] Several villages reacted so negatively when asked to inoculate that they were bypassed entirely.[82] This partly came from the popular belief that physicians introduced plague through the inoculations,[83] something not dissimilar to the idea that COVID-19 was designed to allow Bill Gates to microchip us. We never change.

Because of the challenges of the three *i*'s, other methods were introduced. Rodent control was theoretically an effective method of prevention. However, the absence of inexpensive rodenticides meant that little control was achieved in practice. Western countries had more success because they could rat-proof their grains, storage areas, and silos.[84] Rodent kills reached millions annually but had little impact on the ability of rodents to transmit the disease.[85]

In the array of interventions against the plague, treatment was noticeably absent for the first four decades of the twentieth century.[86] During the Second World War, the antibiotic streptomycin proved to be extremely successful against even the most virulent strains.[87] It was also the first antibiotic used to treat TB,[88] as we'll see in chapter 2. Streptomycin was developed by PhD student Albert Stratz, alongside Elizabeth Bugie, under the supervision of Selman Waksman. Waksman became known as the father of antibiotics and received sole credit for the discovery, including that year's Nobel Prize and significant royalties. Stratz later sued and was given co-credit and royalties[89] but was never able to find work in a top-level microbiology lab thereafter.[90] Streptomycin has been used to treat plague ever since and still remains the drug of choice.[91]

Table 10.1. List of Nobel Prize winners in Physiology or Medicine mentioned in this book

Nobel Prize winners	Year	Discovery
Selman Waksman (with ligitation from Albert Stratz)	1952	Streptomycin, the first antibiotic effective against tuberculosis
Paul Hermann Müller	1948	DDT as a contact poison against several arthropods
Charles Louis Alphonse Laveran	1907	Protozoans as an agent of malaria
Robert Koch	1905	The causative bacillus of tuberculosis
Ronald Ross	1902	Transmission of malaria via mosquitos

Source: Wikipedia.

However, the most decisive breakthrough in plague control also arrived at this time:[92] insecticides, which disrupted transmission by attacking the flea vector.[93] Dichlorodiphenyltrichloroethane (known as DDT) had been developed in 1874 by Othmar Zeidler, an Austrian chemist, but he failed to realize its insecticidal properties.[94] It wasn't until 1939 that the Swiss chemist Paul Hermann Müller found that insects absorbed chemicals differently than mammals. This led him to believe that there were chemicals that were exclusively toxic to insects. He sought to "synthesize the ideal contact insecticide—one which would have a quick and powerful toxic effect upon the largest possible number of insect species while causing little or no harm to plants and warm-blooded animals."[95] He also made it his goal to create an insecticide that was long-lasting, cheap to produce, with a high degree of chemical stability.[96]

In embracing this goal, Müller was motivated by two events. The first of these was a major food shortage in Switzerland, which underscored the need for a better way to control the infestation of crops by insects. The second was the 1918–1922 typhus epidemic in Russia (spread by fleas), which was the most extensive and lethal such epidemic in history.[97]

Tests of DDT by the Swiss government and the United States Department of Agriculture confirmed its effectiveness against the Colorado potato beetle.[98] Further tests demonstrated its effectiveness against a wide range of pests—including the mosquito, louse, flea, and sandfly, which, respectively, spread malaria, typhus, the plague, and various tropical diseases.[99] DDT remained effective for six to eight weeks on interior walls.[100] It lasted twice as long as the next best insecticide and cost three times less.[101] Müller won the Nobel Prize for Medicine in 1948 for these efforts.[102]

DDT was first applied on a large scale in Naples in 1943 by the U.S. Army to combat an outbreak of typhus. Shortly thereafter, it was applied during the bubonic plague epidemic in Dakar, Senegal, in 1944, and against malaria-bearing mosquitoes in Italy.[103] By the 1950s, DDT had become the standard insecticide employed against sporadic outbreaks of bubonic plague and other insect-borne diseases around the world.[104] We'll learn more about the effects of DDT in chapter 1.

The Third Plague was considered active until 1960, when cases dropped below 200 per year.[105] Its disappearance can be attributed to two main factors: improved hygiene and the lack of a present-day animal reservoir for the disease.[106]

Despite eventual control that took nearly a century, further dangers loom. In 1988, scientists at Urnea, in Sweden, succeeded in producing two small genetic mutations in *Y. pseudotuberculosis*; the bacteria became a hundred times more virulent. This led the team to speculate that similar single-point mutations occurring "naturally" in *Y. pestis* might have been the reason for epidemics—in the sense of sudden rises of virulence—of plague among humans in the past.[107] Many low-level diseases can suddenly turn into pandemics,[108] so it is feasible that a fourth plague pandemic could arise in the future. Conversely, similar mutations might also explain the decline of epidemics,[109] much as happened with the Omicron variant of COVID-19.[110]

Once a scourge to millions, bubonic plague is now a treatable disease, with a relatively low case load and very low death rates. Having wreaked havoc on both lives and societies in the past, today it's mostly a mild disease that's easily treatable. As we'll see, that isn't at all the case for many of the diseases in the remainder of the top ten.

Notes

1. C. W. Mcmillen, *Pandemics: A Very Short Introduction* (Oxford: Oxford University Press, 2016).

2. C. Benedict, *Bubonic Plague in Eighteenth-Century China* (Stanford: Stanford University Press, 1996).

3. I. J. Catanach, "The 'Globalization' of Disease? India and the Plague," *Journal of World History* 12, no. 1 (2001): 131–153.

4. R. L. Burrows, "The Third Plague Pandemic and British India: A Transformation of Science, Policy, and Indian Society," *Tenor of Our Times* 10, no. 1 (2021): 127–155.

5. J. Y. Wong et al., "Case Fatality Risk of Influenza A (H1N1pdm09): A Systematic Review," *Epidemiology* 24, no. 6 (2013): 830–841.

6. C. Benedict, "Bubonic Plague in Nineteenth-Century China," *Modern China* 14, no. 2 (1988): 107–155.

7. A. W. Bacot and C. J. Martin, "Observations on the Mechanism of the Transmission of Plague by Fleas," *Journal of Hygiene* 13 (1914): 423–439.

8. C. McEvedy, "The Bubonic Plague," *Scientific American* 258, no. 2 (1988): 118–123.

9. J. D. Forrester et al., "Patterns of Human Plague in Uganda, 2008–2016," *Emerging Infectious Diseases* 23, no. 9 (2017): 1517–1521.

10. J. Piret and G. Boivin, "Pandemics Throughout History," *Frontiers in Microbiology* 11 (2021): 631736.

11. T. V. Inglesby et al., "Plague as a Biological Weapon: Medical and Public Health Management," *Journal of the American Medical Association* 283, no. 17 (2000): 2281–2290.

12. M. Echenberg, "Pestis Redux: The Initial Years of the Third Bubonic Plague Pandemic, 1894–1901," *Journal of World History* 13, no.2 (2002): 429–449.

13. E. G. Pryor, "The Great Plague of Hong Kong," *Journal of the Hong Kong Branch of the Royal Asiatic Society* 15 (1975): 61–70.

14. C. Benedict, *Bubonic Plague in Eighteenth-Century China.*

15. "Association of Schools of Public Health, Weekly Reports for June 15, 1906," *Public Health Reports* 21, no. 24 (1906): 641–672.

16. D. J. Kang, "Bubonic Plague, Western Medicine, and Women: Female Chinese Patients and Colonial Medicine in Hong Kong (1841–1900)," *Research on Women in Modern Chinese History* 26 (2015): 67–132.

17. E. G. Pryor, "The Great Plague of Hong Kong."

18. M. P. Sutphen, "Not What, but Where: Bubonic Plague and the Reception of Germ Theories in Hong Kong and Calcutta, 1894–1897," *Journal of the History of Medicine and Allied Sciences* 52, no. 1 (1997): 81–113.

19. C. Benedict, "Bubonic Plague in Nineteenth-Century China."

20. E. G. Pryor, "The Great Plague of Hong Kong."

21. C. Benedict, "Bubonic Plague in Nineteenth-Century China."

22. A. Starling et al., *Plague, SARS and the Story of Medicine in Hong Kong* (Hong Kong: Hong Kong University Press, 2006).

23. D. J. Kang, "Bubonic Plague."

24. T. Solomon, "Hong Kong, 1894: The Role of James A Lowson in the Controversial Discovery of the Plague Bacillus," *The Lancet* 350, no. 9070 (1997): 59–62.

25. S. Chatterjee, "Plague and Politics in Bengal 1896 to 1898," *Proceedings of the Indian History Congress* 66 (2005): 1194–1201.

26. E. W. Bentley, "The Distribution and Status of *Rattus rattus L.* in the United Kingdom in 1951 and 1956," *The Journal of Animal Ecology* 28, no. 2 (1959): 199–308.

27. M. Echenberg, "Pestis Redux."

28. I. J. Catanach, "Plague and the Tensions of Empire: India, 1896–1918," in *Imperial Medicine and Indigenous Societies*, ed. D. Arnold (Manchester: Manchester University Press, 2017), 149–171.

29. M. Echenberg, "Pestis Redux."

30. I. J. Catanach, "South Asian Muslims and the Plague 1896–c.1914," *South Asia: Journal of South Asian Studies* 22 (1999): 87–107.

31. K. M. Hunter, "Fighting the Bubonic Plague in India," *The Nineteenth Century* 43, no. 256 (1898): 1008–1016.

32. I. J. Catanach, "South Asian Muslims and the Plague 1896–c.1914".

33. A. Proust, *La Défense de l'Europe contre la peste et la Conférence de Venise de 1897* (Paris: Masson, 1897).

34. C. W. McMillen, *Pandemics*.

35. I. J. Catanach, "South Asian Muslims and the Plague 1896–c.1914".

36. K. M. Hunter, "Fighting the Bubonic Plague in India."

37. R. L. Burrows, "The Third Plague Pandemic and British India: A Transformation of Science, Policy, and Indian Society," *Tenor of Our Times* 10, no. 1 (2021): 127–155.

38. R. D. Perry and J.D. Fetherston, "*Yersinia pestis*—Etiologic Agent of Plague," *Clinical Microbiology Reviews* 10, no. 1 (1997): 35–66.

39. M. Echenberg, "Pestis Redux."

40. I. Klein, "Population and Agriculture in Northern India, 1872–1921," *Modern Asian Studies* 8, no. 2 (1974): 191–216.

41. C. Creighton, "Plague in India," *US Government Printing Office* (1907): 309–338.

42. M. Echenberg, "Pestis Redux."

43. E. B. van Heyningen, "Cape Town and the Plague of 1901," *Studies in the History of Cape Town* 4 (1981): 66–107.

44. Maynard Swanson, "The Sanitation Syndrome: Bubonic Plague and Urban Native Policy in the Cape colony, 1900–1909," *Journal of African History* 18, no. 3 (1977): 387–410.

45. P. A. Kalisch, "The Black Death in Chinatown: Plague and Politics in San Francisco 1900–1904," *Arizona and the West* 14, no. 2 (1972): 113–136.

46. G. B. Risse, *Plague, Fear, and Politics in San Francisco's Chinatown* (Baltimore: Johns Hopkins University Press, 2012).

47. J. G. Power, "Media Dependency, Bubonic Plague, and the Social Construction of the Chinese Other," *Journal of Communication Inquiry* 19, no. 1 (1995): 89–110.

48. N. E. Tutorow, "A Tale of Two Hospitals: US Marine Hospital No. 19 and the US Public Health Service Hospital on the Presidio of San Francisco," *California History* 75, no. 2 (1996): 154–169.

49. J. B. Trauner, "The Chinese as Medical Scapegoats in San Francisco, 1870–1905," *California History* 57, no. 1 (1978): 70–87.

50. C. McClain, "Of Medicine, Race, and American Law: The Bubonic Plague Outbreak of 1900," *Law & Social Inquiry* 13, no. 3 (2006): 447–513.

51. N. Wisseman, "'Beware the Yellow Peril and Behold the Black Plague': The Internationalization of American White Supremacy and Its Critiques, Chicago 1919," *Journal of the Illinois State Historical Society* 103, no. 1 (2010): 43–66.

52. V. Liboa, "Brazilian Sanitarian Oswaldo Cruz Faced Three Simultaneous Epidemics," *Agência Brasil* (5 August 2022).

53. D. R. do Nascimento, "The Arrival of the Plague in Sao Paulo in 1899," *Dynamis* 31, no. 1 (2011): 65–83.

54. C. Throp, *The Horrors of the Bubonic Plague* (North Mankate: Capstone Press, 2017).

55. G. Riley, "When the Plague Came to Australia's Shores," *News GP* (23 July 2018).

56. J. A. Thompson, "A Contribution to the Aetiology of Plague," *The Journal of Hygiene* 1, no. 2 (1901): 153–167.

57. H. Sutton, "Ashburton Thompson and the Plague: A Great Epidemiologist and His Triumph over the Black Death," *Journal of the Royal Sanitary Institute* 70, no. 1 (1950): 73–76.

58. M. Echenberg, "Pestis Redux."

59. E. G. Pryor, "The Great Plague of Hong Kong."

60. M. Echenberg, "Pestis Redux."

61. H. P. Williams, "Honolulu's Contention with the Plague," *Boston Herald* (4 March 1900).

62. M. Echenberg, "Pestis Redux."

63. J. C. Mohr, *Plague and Fire: Battling Black Death and the 1900 Burning of Honolulu's Chinatown* (Oxford: Oxford University Press, 2004).

64. M. Echenberg, "Pestis Redux."

65. J.O. Mann, "Plague—Perspectives on a Rare Disease," *Western Journal of Medicine* 140, no. 4 (1984): 650–651.

66. R. Barbieri et al., "*Yersinia pestis*: The Natural History of Plague," *Clinical Microbiology Reviews* 34, no. 1 (2020): e00044–19.

67. K. A. Glatter and P. Finkelman, "History of the Plague: An Ancient Pandemic for the Age of COVID-19," *The American Journal of Medicine* 134, no. 2 (2021): 176–181.

68. D. J. Bibel and T.H. Chen, "Diagnosis of Plague: An Analysis of the Yersin–Kitasato Controversy," *Bacteriological Reviews* 40, no. 3 (1976): 633–651.

69. L. F. Hirst, "Conquest of Plague," *British Medical Journal* 2, no. 4851 (1953): 1432–1433.

70. M. Simond, M.L. Godley, and P.D.E. Mouriquand, "Paul-Louis Simond and His Discovery of Plague Transmission by Rat Fleas: A Centenary," *Journal of the Royal Society of Medicine* 91 (1998): 101–104.

71. R. L. Burrows, "The Third Plague Pandemic."

72. J. Gunter and V. Pandey, "Waldemar Haffkine: The Vaccine Pioneer the World Forgot," *BBC News*, 11 December 2020.

73. J. Busvine, *Disease Transmission by Insects: Its Discovery and 90 Years of Effort to Prevent It* (New York: Springer, 2012).

74. R. L. Burrows, "The Third Plague Pandemic."

75. M. Echenberg, "Pestis Redux."

76. J. Busvine, *Disease Transmission by Insects.*

77. L. E. Quenee and O. Schneewind, "Plague Vaccines and the Molecular Basis of Immunity Against *Yersinia pestis*," *Human Vaccines* 5, no. 12 (2009): 817–823.

78. J. Gunter and V. Pandey, "Waldemar Haffkine."

79. B. J. Hawgood, "Waldemar Mordecai Haffkine, CIE (1860–1930): Prophylactic Vaccination against Cholera and Bubonic Plague in British India," *Journal of Medical Biography* 15, no. 1 (2007): 9–19.

80. J. Gunter and V. Pandey, "Waldemar Haffkine."

81. M. Echenberg, *Plague Ports: The Global Urban Impact of Bubonic Plague, 1894–1901* (New York: New York University Press, 2007).

82. C. Creighton, "Plague in India."

83. W. B. Bannerman, "The Spread of Plague in India," *Epidemiology & Infection* 6, no. 2 (1906): 179–211.

84. J. Busvine, *Disease Transmission by Insects*.

85. L. F. Hirst, "Conquest of Plague."

86. M. Echenberg, "Pestis Redux".

87. K. C. Nicolaou and S. Rigol, "A Brief History of Antibiotics and Select Advances in Their Synthesis," *The Journal of Antibiotics* 71, no. 2 (2018): 153–184.

88. J. F. Murray, D.E. Schraufnagel, and P.C. Hopewell, "Treatment of Tuberculosis: A Historical Perspective," *Annals of the American Thoracic Society* 12, no. 12 (2015): 1749–1759.

89. A. Schatz, E. Bugie, and S. A. Waksman, "Streptomycin, a Substance Exhibiting Antibiotic Activity against Gram-Positive and Gram-Negative Bacteria," *Clinical Orthopaedics and Related Research* 437, no. 1 (2005): 3–6.

90. V. Mistiaen, "Time, and the Great Healer," *The Guardian*, 2 November 2002.

91. R. D. Perry and J. D. Fetherston, "*Yersinia pestis*—Etiologic Agent of Plague".

92. M. Echenberg, "Pestis Redux".

93. J. Busvine, *Disease Transmission by Insects*.

94. D. L. Mulliken, J.D. Zambone, and C.G. Rolph, "DDT: A Persistent Lifesaver," *Natural Resources & Environment* 19 (2004): 3–7.

95. G. A. Matthews, *A History of Pesticides* (Wallingford: CABI, 2018).

96. R. L. Metcalf, "A Century of DDT," *Journal of Agricultural and Food Chemistry* 21, no. 4 (1973): 511–519.

97. S. Henne, "DDT Is still Needed to Fight Malaria," in *Pesticides*, ed. D.A. Miller (Farmington Hills: Greenhaven Press, 2014), 92–100.

98. J. H. Perkins, "Reshaping Technology in Wartime: The Effect of Military Goals on Entomological Research and Insect-Control Practices," *Technology and Culture* 19, no. 2 (1978): 169–186.

99. W. S. Stone, "The Role of DDT in Controlling Insect-Borne Diseases of Man," *Journal of the American Medical Association* 132, no. 9 (1946): 507–509.

100. G. A. Campbell and T. F. West, "Persistence of DDT in Oil-Bound Water-Paint," *Nature* 154, no. 3912 (1944): 512.

101. K. Walker, "Cost-Comparison of DDT and Alternative Insecticides for Malaria Control," *Medical and Veterinary Entomology* 14, no. 4 (2000): 345–354.

102. E. Griswold, "How 'Silent Spring' Ignited the Environmental Movement," *The New York Times*, 21 September 2012.

103. J. Busvine, *Disease Transmission by Insects*.

104. M. Echenberg, "Pestis Redux".

105. J. Frith, "The History of Plague—Part 1: The Three Great Pandemics," *Journal of Military and Veterans' Health* 20, no. 2 (2012): 11–16.

106. B. Bramanti et al., "The Third Plague Pandemic in Europe," *Proceedings of the Royal Society B* 286, no. 1901 (2019): 20182429.

107. R. Rosqvist, M. Skurnik, and H. Wolf-Watz, "Increased Virulence of *Yersinia pseudotuberculosis* by Two Independent Mutations," *Nature* 334 (1988): 522–525.

108. A. T. Tredennick et al., "Anticipating Infectious Disease Re-emergence and Elimination: A Test of Early Warning Signals Using Empirically Based Models," *Journal of the Royal Society Interface* 19, no. 193 (2022): 20220123.

109. R. Rosqvist, M. Skurnik, and H. Wolf-Watz, "Increased Virulence of *Yersinia pseudotuberculosis*."

110. C. Del Rio and P. N. Malani, "COVID-19 in 2022—The Beginning of the End or the End of the Beginning?," *Journal of the American Medical Association* 327, no. 24 (2022): 2389–2390.

9 Cocoliztli

I n 1519, when the Spanish arrived in mainland Mexico (then called New Spain), the Mexican population was estimated at 15–30 million people; by the end of the century, only 2 million people lived in the country.[1] What happened to wipe out 93% of the population in just 81 years?

For historical context, we need to talk about some other diseases first. On the other side of the world, syphilis was first recorded in 1495 in Italy, when the French king Charles VIII invaded Naples.[2] Since this was only two years after Columbus had returned from the Americas, considerable debate has raged as to whether Columbus brought the disease to Europe from the New World or if it had simply not been previously recognized.[3] Paleopathologic studies of skeletons of Native Americans who died before Columbus's arrival suggest evidence of syphilis-like diseases in the New World, with cases dating from 7000 years ago.[4] However, as recently as 2020, it was finally shown that diverse syphilis strains were circulating in Europe decades before Columbus left.[5]

If Europeans thought Columbus had brought outbreaks like syphilis back from the New World, the reverse was certainly true. A great many diseases were inflicted on the native peoples of the Americas, including smallpox, chickenpox, measles, and mumps.[6] Smallpox was particularly virulent for indigenous Americans, including the Aztecs, because they'd never been exposed to the virus and thus possessed no natural immunity.[7]

It's instructive to ask what the Spanish were even doing in Mexico at this time. European colonization was under way in force, but that itself has its roots in another disease that makes an appearance in the top ten.

Between September 1520 and August 1521, the indigenous populations were decimated by an outbreak of smallpox[8] that killed some eight million people.[9] We'll revisit smallpox in chapter 3; this devastating epidemic is just setting the scene for the Mexican epidemics to come in the sixteenth century. Having lost a sizable percentage of their population to smallpox, the native inhabitants of Mexico could hardly have been braced for an entirely different epidemic to come their way a generation later.

The cocoliztli epidemic of 1545–1548 killed between *7 and 17 million* people, who died from Mexican haemorrhagic fever.[10] This was an estimated 45% of the entire population—many of whom were either survivors of the smallpox epidemic or their children.[11] Severe droughts extending across Mexico interacted with ecologic and sociologic conditions, magnifying the impact of the disease and causing severe population collapse.[12] This was the worst of three major epidemics in Mexico that century, with the smallpox outbreak preceding it and another haemorrhagic-fever epidemic following a few decades later.[13] *Cocoliztli* is a native Mexican word, originating from the Nahuatl language, usually translated as "pestilence" but more accurately as "pustules."[14]

The symptoms were described at the time by Franciscan Friar Juan de Torquemada thusly:

> The fevers were contagious, burning, and continuous, all of them pestilential, in most part lethal. The tongue was dry and black. Enormous thirst. Urine of the colors sea-green, vegetal-green, and black, sometimes passing from the greenish color to the pale. Pulse was frequent, fast, small, and weak—sometimes even null. The eyes and the whole body were yellow. This stage was followed by delirium and seizures. Then, hard and painful nodules appeared behind one or both ears along with heartache, chest pain, abdominal pain, tremor, great anxiety, and dysentery.[15]

The progress of the disease was fast: from the onset of symptoms, the disease ran its course in only three or four days, usually concluding in the victim's death. By the second or third day, it was said the sufferer broke down mentally, going sometimes entirely insane.[16]

Treatments for cocoliztli were rudimentary and primarily focused on stopping the dysentery, attempting to staunch the bloody flux and letting the purulent fluid out of the nodules behind the ears.[17] This suggests that physicians of the time who were dealing with this epidemic were still operating under the Hippocratic theory of the four humours. The humours were thought to be the chemical systems regulating human behaviour. Hippocrates then applied this idea to medicine, suggesting that illness came from an excess or deficiency in any of the four humours: blood, black bile, yellow bile, and phlegm.[18] Blood was believed to be produced exclusively by the liver and associated with a sanguine nature; an excess of yellow bile was thought to produce aggression; too much black bile secreted by the spleen caused melancholy or gloomy temperaments; while phlegm was associated with passive behaviour.[19] Treatment of diseases involved restoring the balance if there was too much of one or more of these humours.[20] This idea fell out of favour in the 1850s with the advent of germ theory, which showed that many diseases previously thought to be caused by the humours were in fact a result of pathogens.[21]

Using dendrochronological evidence (from tree rings), it's been shown that outbreaks of cocoliztli consistently occurred after periods of severe drought.[22] However, there were other peculiarities of its spread that could not as easily be accounted for. For example, it appeared to infect and kill younger people at a greater rate than older people, which seems counterintuitive. Most diseases (e.g., COVID-19) wreak greater havoc on the weak or elderly than on the young and healthy.[23] The exceptions to this tend to be diseases where some pre-existing immunity is present, perhaps from a previous outbreak that gave the older generations some protection.[24] This disease affected regions where the predominant population was native Mexican, only attacking the Spaniards much later.[25] This suggests that the disease may have been a known European infection which the Spanish brought with them.

Association with droughts could suggest a zoonosis* of rodents; droughts and rainfalls are influential in the epidemiology of hanta-like viruses, leptospirosis, and other diseases. Hantavirus is a pulmonary disease carried by rodents, with infection being passed to humans almost exclusively through rodent excrement,[26] though human-to-human transmission occurred in South America in 2005 and 2019.[27] It's also entirely possible that something more familiar may have had unusual manifestations in an immune-naïve and malnourished population.

As devastating as the mid-century outbreak was, it wasn't the last cocoliztli outbreak to afflict Mexico in the sixteenth century. A generation later, in June 1576, haemorrhagic fever returned and decimated the remaining populations. Torquemada was also a witness to the devastation wrought by this later epidemic: "In the year 1576 a great mortality and pestilence that lasted for more than a year overcame the Indians. It was so big that it ruined and destroyed almost the entire land. The place we know as New Spain was left almost empty."[28] Indeed, the 60,000-strong city of Tepeaca lost 86% of its citizens. Cholula saw a decline from 15,000 inhabitants to 9,000 with a 40% death rate. Nochistlan suffered a 67% loss in its inhabitants as a result of the disease. The overall mortality caused by this epidemic was a loss of about 2 million people from the country's by-then 4.4 million.[29] The net result of these two epidemics and the smallpox one that preceded them was, as we have noted, a population crash of 85%–93% throughout the sixteenth century.

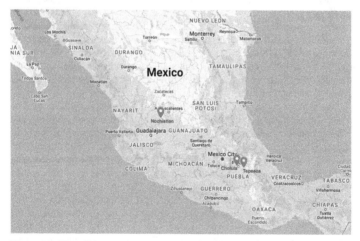

Figure 9.1. Map of Mexico showing Nochistlan (west), Cholula (closest to Mexico City), and Tepeaca (east).

Source: Google Maps.

Both cocoliztli epidemics started in the northern and central Mexican Highlands and spread from there; cocoliztli remained rare in the warm

---

* A zoonotic disease is one that has passed from animals to humans and can do so again.

lowland areas of the Gulf of Mexico and the Pacific coast. This suggests that mosquitoes were not the vector, since they prefer lowlands.[30]

The 1576–1580 epidemic marked a turning point in the development of Mexican culture and of Spanish/Indian relations. Life for the dwindling native population became far more difficult, as the Spanish regime, accustomed to the once-abundant pool of native labour, sought to maintain tribute payments and tax revenues at their former levels by increasingly coercive means. In many areas, the towns and villages recently built in anticipation of a brighter future were simply abandoned as their populations withered away, the landscape of pyramids and temple platforms replaced by hundreds of churches.[31]

Beyond these two major outbreaks, eleven more outbreaks of cocoliztli were reported, lasting throughout the first half of the seventeenth century. They occurred in 1555, 1559, 1566, 1587–1588, 1592–1593, 1601–1602, 1604–1607, 1613, 1624–1631, 1633–1634, and 1641–1642,[32] but information about them is scarce. Recent investigations concluded that the deaths of so many indigenous people may have altered Earth's climate, as no one was left to tend land and till fields, so vegetation reclaimed huge expanses previously used for agriculture. This depleted carbon dioxide from the atmosphere, which contributed to the "Little Ice Age" of 1650.[33]

Cocoliztli has similar characteristics to the haemorrhagic variant of Ebola.[34] Indeed, the nature of the disease remained a mystery for a very long time, with a long list of hypothesized diseases being suggested, including typhus, pneumonic plague, leptospirosis, measles, dengue, hantavirus, yellow fever, and malaria.[35] However, none quite matched, so it was long thought to be an unspecified (possibly long-eradicated) viral haemorrhagic fever.[36]

Viruses are biological entities that infect cells and replicate themselves. Outside the cell, viruses exist as free particles called virions, which are typically RNA or DNA genomes surrounded by a protein shell called a capsid.* Viruses differ from other life forms by the fact that the virions are disassembled during their intercellular, replicative phase.[37]

We'll cover some of these more well-known diseases in this book, but it's worth discussing a few of the others. Viral haemorrhagic fevers vary from uniformly severe infections, with case-fatality rates greater than 60% (e.g., filoviruses), to mostly asymptomatic infections,† wherein a minority of infected individuals develop haemorrhagic fever (e.g., yellow fever and dengue).[38] Ebola is the most famous today, thanks to multiple ongoing outbreaks of recent years, and is spread from human to human—including from dead bodies, often during funeral rites—through direct contact with bodily fluids.[39] Individuals begin to experience an onset of symptoms, including headaches, vomiting, loss of appetite, diarrhoea, stomach pains, lethargy, aching muscles or joints, and difficulties swallowing and breathing, in addition to unexplained bleeding.[40] Following this, symptoms further progress to weakened liver and kidney functions, in addition to more serious haemorrhagic symptoms such as internal and external bleeding.[41] Upon developing these symptoms, infected individuals can spread the virus to others. Individuals who

---

* A genome is the complete set of genetic material in an organism.

† Asymptomatic infections are those that do not present symptoms in the infected individual but are transmissible to others.

develop Ebola virus disease usually die within about 10 days from the onset of the illness.[42]

The other (mostly haemorrhagic) diseases that were postulated as the source of cocoliztli read like a who's who of tropical infections. Typhus is a disease caused by bacteria usually carried by fleas, mites, lice, or ticks. Epidemic typhus wreaks particular havoc on people in poor, crowded, and unsanitary conditions.[43] Leptospirosis is one of the most geographically widespread zoonoses in the world, with greater incidence in tropical regions;[44] pulmonary haemorrhage is a major, often lethal, manifestation of leptospirosis, the pathogenesis of which remains unclear.[45]

Attempts have been made to weaponize various haemorrhagic fever viruses—including Ebola, Marburg, Lassa, Machupo, and Junin viruses—both in the former Soviet Union during the Cold War and in the United States prior to the abolishment of its biological warfare program in 1969.[46] Aum Shinrikyo, the Japanese cult responsible for the 1995 sarin gas attack on the Tokyo subway that killed 12 people,[47] attempted to acquire Ebola virus.[48] An antiviral drug against haemorrhagic fever was recently developed in the Scientific Research Institute of Military Medicine in Saint Petersburg, Russia, with likely collaboration with North Korea, as part of a bioweapons research program.[49]

The cause of cocoliztli has only recently been pinpointed as a form of *Salmonella*, although different to the food-poisoning kind most people are familiar with today. Non-typhoid *Salmonella* figures prominently as the leading cause of bacterial foodborne disease,[50] in part because of its ability to adapt to environmental changes.[51] Symptoms include spiking fever and abdominal cramps coupled with underlying bacteremia in the first week of disease, with watery diarrhoea (or constipation) and persistent abdominal pain in the second week of illness.[52]

The type of *Salmonella* that appears to have caused cocoliztli was not definitively linked to the epidemic until 2018. A team looked at skeletons in a Mexican cemetery during the first cocoliztli epidemic and found *Salmonella paratyphi C* (SpC) DNA in 10 out of 29 dental samples; this DNA was identical to that in an 800-year-old skeleton found in Norway.[53] There was no evidence of this DNA in skeletons in the same cemetery that predated the epidemic;[54] suggesting that this was a new infection brought over from Europe.

Debate has arisen as to whether the *Salmonella* link is conclusive. Some of the arguments against it as a cause of cocoliztli include a lack of prodromal period* (SpC has a prodromal period of a week); rapid death (SpC takes three to four weeks to kill a host and is only fatal in about 40% of cases); bleeding (not a common feature of SpC); and the lack of cocoliztli in coastal areas (imported diseases would have been present in ports).[55] However, all other known candidates have been eliminated, suggesting that cocoliztli was either a disease that has since vanished—despite the fact that diseases almost never disappear on their own; they usually go quiescent in reservoir populations and re-emerge later or remain at low levels—or was a variant of something we know, with SpC the most likely candidate.[56]

---

* The prodromal period is the time between the initial appearance of symptoms and the full development of a rash or fever.

Today, the Centers for Disease Control and Prevention estimate enteric fever–causing *Salmonella* results in more than 21 million cases globally and about 5,700 illnesses in the United States every year.[57] However, modern medicine can handle this easily; treatment with antimicrobial agents has reduced the case-fatality rate to less than 1%, although resistance to drugs is emerging.[58] Whether cocoliztli is this type of *Salmonella* or a now-vanished disease, this is another example of a disease that has essentially come and gone, wreaking its havoc before succumbing to science. Unfortunately, that's not true for the next disease.

Notes

1. S. F. Cook and L. B. Simpson, "The Population of Central Mexico in the Sixteenth Century," *Ibero Americana* 31 (1948): 43–55.
2. C. Quetel, *The History of Syphilis* (Baltimore: Johns Hopkins Press, 1990).
3. B. M. Rothschild, "History of Syphilis," *Clinical Infectious Diseases* 40 (2005): 1454–1463.
4. D. Farhi and N. Dupin, "Origins of Syphilis and Management in the Immunocompetent Patient: Facts and Controversies," *Clinics in Dermatology* 28, no. 5 (2010): 533–538.
5. K. Majander et al., "Ancient Bacterial Genomes Reveal a High Diversity of *Treponema pallidum* Strains in Early Modern Europe," *Current Biology* 30, no. 19 (2020): 3788–3803.
6. A. I. Qureshi, "Ebola Virus Disease Epidemic in Light of Other Epidemics," *Ebola Virus Disease* (2016): 39–65.
7. R. Gunderman, "How Smallpox Devastated the Aztecs—and Helped Spain Conquer an American Civilization 500 Years Ago," *The Conversation*, 19 February 2019.
8. M. Verza, "500 Years Ago, another Epidemic Swept Mexico: Smallpox," *AP News*, 28 September 2020.
9. N. Lloyd, "Cocolitzi: The Mystery Pestilence," *Historical Blindness* podcast, 18 May 2020.
10. R. Acuña-Soto et al., "When Half of the Population Died: The Epidemic of Hemorrhagic Fevers of 1576 in Mexico," *FEMS Microbiology Letters* 240 (2004): 1–5.
11. A. Chen, "One of History's Worst Epidemics May Have Been Caused by a Common Microbe," *Science* (16 January 2018).
12. R. Acuña-Soto et al., "When Half of the Population Died: The Epidemic of Hemorrhagic Fevers of 1576 in Mexico."
13. R. Acuña-Soto et al., "Megadrought and Megadeath in 16th Century Mexico," *Emerging Infectious Diseases* 8 (2002): 360–362.
14. C. Dodds Pennock, "Have Scientists Really Found the Germ Responsible for Killing 15m Aztecs?," *The Conversation*, 18 January 2018.
15. S. Zhang, "A New Clue to the Mystery Disease that once Killed Most of Mexico," *The Atlantic*, 15 January 2018.
16. N. Lloyd, "Cocolitzi: The Mystery Pestilence."
17. N. Lloyd, "Cocolitzi: The Mystery Pestilence."
18. W. A. Jackson, "A Short Guide to Humoral Medicine," *Trends in Pharmacological Sciences* 22 (2001): 487–489.
19. L. A. Clark and D. Watson, "Temperament: An Organizing Paradigm for Trait Psychology," in *Handbook of Personality: Theory and Research*, ed. O.P. John, R.W. Robins, and L. W. Pervin (New York: Guilford Press, 2008), 265–286.

20. W. Bynum, "Epidemiology: The History of Disease and Epidemics," *Science Focus* (8 April 2020).

21. F. Lagay, "The Legacy of Humoral Medicine," *Virtual Mentor* 4, no. 7 (2002): 206–208.

22. R. Acuña-Soto et al., "Megadrought and Megadeath in 16th Century Mexico."

23. D. Cortis, "On Determining the Age Distribution of COVID-19 Pandemic," *Frontiers in Public Health* 8 (2020): 202.

24. M. Lemaitre and F. Carrat, "Comparative Age Distribution of Influenza Morbidity and Mortality During Seasonal Influenza Epidemics and the 2009 H1N1 Pandemic," *BMC Infectious Diseases* 10, no. 1 (2010): 1–5.

25. N. Lloyd, "Cocolitzi: The Mystery Pestilence."

26. C. B. Jonsson, L. T. Figueiredo, and O. Vapalahti, "A Global Perspective on Hantavirus Ecology, Epidemiology, and Disease," *Clinical Microbiology Reviews* 23, no. 2 (2010): 412–441.

27. V. P. Martinez et al., "Person-to-Person Transmission of Andes Virus," *Emerging Infectious Diseases* 11, no. 12 (2005): 1848–1853.

28. A. H. Rajagopalan, *Portraying the Aztec Past: The Codices Boturini, Azcatitlan, and Aubin* (Austin: University of Texas Press, 2018).

29. R. Acuña-Soto, L. C. Romero, and J. H. Maguire, "Large Epidemics of Hemorrhagic Fevers in Mexico 1545–1815," *American Journal of Tropical Medicine and Hygiene* 62, no. 6 (2000): 733–739.

30. D. Garner, "Coco-whatzi?," *Microbiology Nuts and Bolts* (24 September 2020).

31. J. S. Marr and J. B. Kiracofe, "Was the Huey Cocoliztli a Haemorrhagic Fever?," *Medical History* 44, no. 3 (2000): 341–362.

32. R. Acuña-Soto, L. C. Romero, and J. H. Maguire, "Large Epidemics of Hemorrhagic Fevers in Mexico 1545–1815."

33. A. Koch et al., "Earth System Impacts of the European Arrival and Great Dying in the Americas after 1492," *Quaternary Science Reviews* 207 (2019): 13–36.

34. A. I. Qureshi, "Ebola Virus Disease Epidemic in light of Other Epidemics."

35. Å. J. Vågene et al., "*Salmonella enterica* Genomes from Victims of a Major Sixteenth-Century Epidemic in Mexico," *Nature Ecology & Evolution* 2, no. 3 (2018): 520–528.

36. R. Acuña-Soto et al., "Megadrought and Megadeath in 16th Century Mexico."

37. M. Breitbart and F. Rohwer, "Here a Virus, There a Virus, Everywhere the Same Virus?," *Trends in Microbiology* 13, no. 6 (2005): 278–284.

38. S. Paessler and D. H. Walker, "Pathogenesis of the Viral Hemorrhagic Fevers," *Annual Review of Pathology: Mechanisms of Disease* 8 (2013): 411–440.

39. D. J. Funk and A. Kumar, "Ebola Virus Disease: an Update for Anesthesiologists and Intensivists," *Canadian Journal of Anaesthesia* 62 (2014): 80–91.

40. B. Alyward et al., "Ebola Virus Disease in West Africa—the First 9 Months of the Epidemic and Forward Projections," *New England Journal of Medicine* 371 (2014): 1481–1495.

41. World Health Organization, "Ebola Virus Disease Fact Sheet," 23 February 2021, http://www.who.int/mediacentre/factsheets/fs103/en/ (accessed 2 June 2022).

42. G. Chowell and H. Nishiura, "Transmission Dynamics and Control of Ebola Virus Disease (EVD): A Review," *BMC Medicine* 12, article 196 (2014).

43. D. Raoult, T. Woodward, and J.S. Dumler, "The History of Epidemic Typhus," *Infectious Disease Clinics of North America* 18, no. 1 (2004): 127–140.

44. P. N. Levett et al., "Two Methods for Rapid Serological Diagnosis of Acute Leptospirosis," *Clinical and Diagnostic Laboratory Immunology* 8, no. 2 (2001): 349–351.

45. A. R. Bharti et al., "Leptospirosis: A Zoonotic Disease of Global Importance," *The Lancet Infectious Diseases* 3, no. 12 (2003): 757–771.

46. D. G. Bausch and C. J. Peters, "The Viral Hemorrhagic Fevers," in *Beyond Anthrax: The Weaponization of Infectious Diseases*, ed. L.I. Lutwick and S.M. Lutwick (Totowa: Humana Press, 2009), 107–144.

47. R. Schroëder, *The History of Cults: From the Satanic Sects to the Manson Family* (London: Carlton Books, 2019).

48. S. Stewart, "Evaluating Ebola as a Biological Weapon," *Forbes* (27 October 2014).

49. D. Shoham and Z. E. Wolfson, "The Russian Biological Weapons Program: Vanished or Disappeared?," *Critical Reviews in Microbiology* 30, no.4 (2004): 241–261.

50. J. Y. D'Aoust, "Salmonella and the International Food Trade," *International Journal of Food Microbiology* 24, no. 1–2 (1994): 11–31.

51. T. Humphrey, "Salmonella, Stress Responses and Food Safety," *Nature Reviews Microbiology* 2, no. 6 (2004): 504–509.

52. J. Y. D'Aoust, "Salmonella and the International Food Trade."

53. Z. Zhou et al., "Pan-Genome Analysis of Ancient and Modern *Salmonella enterica* Demonstrates Genomic Stability of the Invasive para C Lineage for Millennia," *Current Biology* 28, no. 15 (2018): 2420–2428.

54. S. Zhang, "A New Clue to the Mystery Disease that once Killed Most of Mexico."

55. D. Garner, "Coco-whatzi?"

56. N. Varlik, "How Do Pandemics End? History Suggests Diseases Fade but Are Almost never Truly Gone," *The Conversation* (14 October 2020).

57. Centers for Disease Control and Prevention, *Typhoid Fever and Paratyphoid Fever*, https://www.cdc.gov/typhoid-fever/sources.html (accessed 2 June 2022).

58. V. Manchanda, "Treatment of Enteric Fever in Children on the Basis of Current Trends of Antimicrobial Susceptibility of Salmonella enterica serovar typhi and paratyphi A," *Indian Journal of Medical Microbiology* 24, no. 2 (2006): 101.

8 HIV/AIDS

Most diseases are old. HIV/AIDS is new. Where most other serious pandemics arise out of existing diseases or mutations from them, HIV/AIDS not only arose in a new way, it also went on to become extremely widespread in a remarkably short span of time.

AIDS (acquired immunodeficiency syndrome) was first identified in late 1980, when a series of apparently unrelated illnesses among gay men in New York and San Francisco were understood to result from a weakened immune system.[1] This disease was originally called GRID (gay-related immune deficiency)[2] and nicknamed "the gay plague," as it was initially seen by Western medical systems in sexually active gay men.[3]

The viral cause of AIDS was identified as HIV (human immunodeficiency virus) in 1983[4] and by this time was understood to infect more than just gay men.[5] However, the primary subpopulations who were infected belonged to the "four *h*'s": homosexuals, haemophiliacs,* heroin users, and Haitians.[6] Tainted blood supplies meant people were infected through blood transfusions;[7] sharing of needles was an efficient method of disease spread;[8] and the disease—like most infections—ravaged the poor.[9]

Women were initially thought immune to the disease, the thinking being that the "rugged vagina" could take a lot of punishment, unlike the "vulnerable rectum"[10] (ignoring the fact that many women also engage in anal sex);[11] medical advice to women who had bisexual male partners was to not worry about a supposedly "male" disease, which caused a lot of women to become infected unecessarily.[12]

Stereotyping around the infected subpopulations caused the disease to go unrecognized for a long time in the general population. It was a disease that affected unloved people doing unloved things that mainstream society absolutely did not want to discuss. If you were going to design the perfect disease to target the weak spots in our society, HIV would be it.

Famously, Ronald Reagan was almost completely silent on the subject of AIDS, despite being U.S. president from 1980 through 1988, key years of the AIDS crisis.[13] Many of Reagan's advisors were startlingly unsympathetic to the plight of the nation's thousands of AIDS victims; his surgeon general, C. Everett Koop, explained that Reagan's closest advisors "took the stand, 'They are only getting what they justly deserve.'"[14]

---

* Haemophilia is a blood disorder in which the blood does not clot properly.

In part, this was because of a Republican backlash to a pandemic that occurred in 1976. When there was an outbreak of swine flu, President Gerald Ford mobilized government to vaccinate Americans in unprecedented numbers.[15] However, a rash of Guillain–Barré syndrome—there were 362 cases in the six weeks following the immunization of 45 million people, an 8.8-fold increase over the background rate, although the link remains unproven—caused the program to be suspended.[16] The backlash was considerable, contributing in part to the Republican loss of the presidency in 1976,[17] although hindsight has claimed it was perhaps the finest hour of America's public-health bureaucracy.[18] Disease management has never been part of a Republican platform since.

Since 1980, AIDS has killed *36 million* people.[19] While the initial Western diagnoses were among gay men, the vast majority of those afflicted have been in sub-Saharan Africa, where the disease is spread primarily through heterosexual sex. Other methods of spread, such as needle sharing, blood transfusions, or mother-to-child transmission have largely been eliminated, thanks to improved screening practices, needle-sharing programs, and treatment during childbirth, leaving sexual transmission as the leading cause of new infections.[20]

HIV acts by attacking the immune system, specifically the memory $CD4^+$ T cells (although it attacks other cells too).[21] These cells are responsible for forming memory of previous infections and communicating between the two major branches of the immune system:[22] B cells create antibodies to fight off new infections, while T cells destroy infected cells in order to shut down virus-making machinery.[23] However, without the ability to communicate between the two branches, the immune system is hobbled.[24] If you were going to design the perfect disease to target the weak spots in our immune system, HIV would be it.

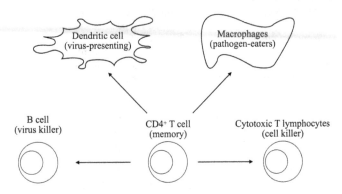

Figure 8.1. Schematic diagram showing the role that $CD4^+$ T cells play in the immune system.

Source: Created by the author.

However, this attack takes time. The virus itself is fast, with a viral half-life of around two days,[25] meaning it takes that long for the initial amount of virus to be halved. Half-life is a measure of decay, because tracking individual virus particles is difficult and imprecise, whereas tracking the *rate* of reduction is much more reliable.[26] Two days isn't long at all, which means there's a very fast turnaround: an individual virus particle has to infect a new cell pretty quickly, so it had better make a lot of new offspring in order to stay viable. The virus acts in the opposite way to the usual method (it uses RNA to create DNA), so it's known as a retrovirus.[27]

Despite the fast rate of viral decay, it takes many years for the immune system to be sufficiently weakened to trip the AIDS threshold. During this time, infected people have no symptoms, which—in the absence of testing—allows the disease to spread unchecked for many years. Because of the very short half-life but long quiescent period, viral particles present in the body a decade after infection are several thousand generations removed from the original virus. In this time, the virus can undergo as much genetic change as humans might experience in the course of millions of years.[28] About a decade after infection, people die of "opportunistic infections": those otherwise benign diseases that the weakened immune system cannot fight off.[29] It follows that the immune system is fighting off diseases all the time; it deals with many infections quietly and efficiently, with only the few failures the ones that we see.[30] However, without the CD4⁺ T cells, infections that would usually be dealt with easily are suddenly able to take hold.[31]

Although the epidemic exploded during the 1980s—there were 159 AIDS cases in the United States in 1981 and 117,508 in 1989—historians have examined possible circulation before this time.[32] For people to show symptoms in 1981, the disease must have been widely circulating in the 1970s, but there are confirmed cases in Haiti in 1966,[33] with the earliest known case an HIV-positive man who died in the Democratic Republic of Congo in 1959.[34]

The origins of HIV/AIDS are murky and shrouded in controversy. HIV jumped species from chimpanzees, gorillas, and macaques, sometime before 1910.[35] These primates develop SIV (simian immunodeficiency virus)[36] and sometimes AIDS, but for the most part the infection doesn't harm or kill the animal.[37] The chimpanzee and gorilla strains led to HIV-1, which is the more common and more lethal strain,[38] while the rhesus macaque version is very similar to HIV-2, which is largely confined to sub-Saharan Africa and is less lethal[39] (not everyone with HIV-2 progresses to AIDS).

Precisely how the virus jumped species is unknown, but it appears to have done so independently at least four times;[40] there is no evidence that this happened as a result of human–primate sexual relations, as has sometimes been claimed.[41] Based on the biology of the virus, transmission must have occurred through cutaneous or mucous membrane exposure to infected ape blood and/or body fluids. Such exposures occur most commonly in the context of bushmeat hunting.[42] Unfortunately, we may never have a definitive answer.

By 1920, the disease had made its way to Léopoldville,* the capital of the Democratic Republic of the Congo, and then made its way through Africa along increasingly developing transportation networks.[43] Polio vaccines were incubated in primate serum (as was common) during a polio vaccination campaign in the Democratic Republic of the Congo, Burundi, and Rwanda

---

* Now called Kinshasa.

in 1957–1960, which may have inadvertently spread the disease even fur-ther.[44] Female sex workers were treated for syphilis using non-sterile needles in the 1950s and 1960s, coinciding with an explosion in sex work as migration and unemployment rates skyrocketed; Haitians employed by various United Nations agencies in Africa migrated back and forth, taking the disease with them.[45] These various routes explain why the disease appeared simultane-ously in multiple locations, rather than spreading from a point source.

The epidemic wrought massive devastation on lives and economies in the developing world in particular. South Africa was at one point on track for economic collapse solely as a result of HIV/AIDS.[46] AIDS took out a large swath of a generation of otherwise able-bodied workers and parents, leaving behind an orphan crisis[47] and a severe shortage of people to care for the sick.[48] Death became so routine in South Africa that the coffin industry became a major source of economic tension.[49] Being thin was a sign of illness, so fat bodies were fetishized,[50] and there was a massive rise in child-headed households in which the main caregiver was younger than 18.[51]

Myths around diseases have flourished since time immemorial, because humans are very good at telling stories, whether or not those stories are based on fact. In the nineteenth century, harmful myths grew around syph-ilis, gonorrhea, and other STIs, with perhaps the worst being that you could cure them by having sex with a virgin. (Note: you can't.) A descendent of this same Victorian-era myth—likely thanks to colonialism—found its way to Africa by the end of the twentieth century.[52] How do you ensure that your sexual partner is a virgin? Sadly, the answer was to have sex with babies,[53] something that happened far too frequently. Another myth was one claimed by Thabo Mbeki, then-president of South Africa, who claimed that HIV did not cause AIDS, instead suggesting a variety of herbal remedies to treat the virus; a Harvard-led study estimated that this myth caused 330,000 pre-ventable deaths.[54]

Fears of the disease weren't just about death, however. AIDS is a lingering illness, leading to a wasting away over a long period of time.[55] Symptoms include rapid weight loss; recurring fever or profuse night sweats; fatigue; prolonged swelling of the lymph glands in the armpits, groin, or neck; diar-rhoea; sores of the mouth, anus, or genitals; pneumonia; blotches on or under the skin or inside the mouth, nose, or eyelids; memory loss; depression; and other neurologic disorders.[56] This is why the DALYs for HIV/AIDS (mentioned in the introduction) are so high: there's the number of deaths but also the (many) years of healthy life lost because of the disease.

It was originally thought that an effective vaccine would be developed against the virus,[57] but this has proven elusive in the 40 years since its identification.[58] Vaccine development for HIV is big business, averaging $800 million per year, but there has been very little progress.[59] An HIV vaccine was developed in 2009, but it was not approved, as its efficacy was just 31%,[60] meaning that more than two thirds of those vaccinated would lack protection against infection.

The HIV epidemic appeared just after the gay-rights movement of the 1970s, when lesbians and gay men organized to raise awareness and form communities; these structures allowed the community to mobilize far more effectively around HIV/AIDS than might otherwise have happened.[61] One of the more notable results of this community building was the formation of ACT UP: a street protest group that demanded—and eventually got—treatment for HIV/AIDS.[62] Activism around AIDS was a prime force in introducing living wills, health care proxies, do-not-resuscitate orders, and hospice care into common parlance.[63]

While vaccine development floundered, treatment progressed in fits and starts. Antiretroviral therapy was first developed in 1987. A drug called azidothymidine (AZT) was originally developed for cancer, but it was found to work against HIV, in one of those serendipitous breakthroughs that science is famous for.[64] After it was discovered that nearly all avian cancers were caused by retroviruses, AZT was developed but proved to be biologically inert in mice. When HIV was discovered to be a retrovirus, about 10 years later, AZT was dusted off and found to be effective. It works by blocking the transcription of the viral RNA onto DNA, thus stopping a cell from creating new virus.[65] AZT did what it needed to in the extremely sick, bringing patients back from death's door to a much healthier state, for a while. However, the side effects were horrendous, and the long-term prognosis was not good for those who had HIV but not AIDS.[66] Chemotherapy just isn't a good preventative tactic.

Ecological theory suggests that all species (even quasi-species like viruses, which aren't quite alive but have some characteristics in common with life, such as replication) can be broken down into two fundamental camps: lions or rabbits. The lioness expends a lot of effort making a very sophisticated offspring, but she doesn't make very many of them. The rabbit strategy is to make as many offspring as possible, in the hope that enough of them survive. Neither strategy is inherently better than the other (it depends on circumstances and the environment), but there's a clear division.[67]

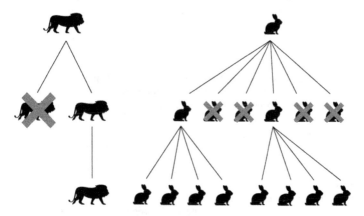

Figure 8.2. Lions vs. rabbits strategy.
Source: Created by the author.

HIV is very clearly following the rabbit strategy. (That's not true of all viruses; measles is very successful, but it has a lion strategy.) Each HIV virus results in the creation of a very large number of offspring, but most are not viable. HIV is an RNA virus, meaning it's much simpler than most other viruses. It needs DNA to replicate, but it uses the machinery of the host cell to transcribe its RNA into DNA.[68] Unlike COVID-19 (itself another RNA virus),[69] HIV lacks an error-checking capability that ensures the daughter viruses look like the mother, correcting errors in the DNA if necessary.[70] Instead, HIV simply creates a huge number of offspring, in the hope that enough will be viable. The average HIV-positive individual produces up to a billion virus particles *per day*.[71] This is what makes finding a cure so difficult. If any evolutionary pressure is applied (such as a vaccine or treatment), the chances of a mutant virus emerging are very high indeed.

Most mutants pay a cost for their evolutionary advantage; to expend energy getting around the pressure of a drug or vaccine, they need to make sacrifices elsewhere, often in their transmissibility.[72] If the drug were not present, the wild-type strain (i.e., the strain most suited to survival in the absence of such pressure) would reassert itself, assuming it still exists.[73] However, the trade-off when the drug is present is more than adequate to give the mutant an advantage. This drug-resistant strain can then be transmitted to someone else, who may have no wild-type strain to out-compete it. As a result, the drugs can fail from the outset.[74]

Other, more effective, drugs with a similar mechanism to AZT have since been developed, collectively called reverse transcriptase inhibitors. A second class of drugs with an entirely different mechanism were later developed: protease inhibitors allow only non-viable new virus to be created, although the cell is destroyed in the process.[75] A third class called entry inhibitors were designed based on lessons learned from the Black Death (more on that in chapter 5).

Since the probability of a chance mutation to a single drug was extremely high, mathematicians reasoned that a combination of two drugs might be better.[76] It was, but not enough; the probability of a mutation that just happened to resist both drugs was still unacceptably high.[77] However, these probabilities decrease significantly as the number of drugs increase, and the mathematicians realized that the crucial number of drugs was three: the probability of a chance mutation to all three drugs was vanishingly small.[78] Suddenly, in December 1995, we had a treatment that worked: the triple-drug cocktail.[79]

Fifteen years after HIV was first seen, there was a life-saving measure that could bring patients with AIDS back to a functioning immune system and keep them there. AIDS was no longer a death sentence, but rather a disease you could live with. Triple-drug therapy isn't a cure—the virus hides in any number of places that the drugs can't reach, so if you stop treatment, the viral load quickly rebounds—but regular pills can keep the disease at bay, giving millions of HIV-positive people the chance of living a full life.[80] Taken properly (with greater than 95% adherence), the drugs keep the virus below detectable level, which means that the chances of transmission to a seronegative partner are exceedingly small, even without condoms.[81]

Of course, the existence of a lifelong treatment doesn't automatically mean everyone has access to it. For one thing, the treatment was set at U.S. drug prices, costing more than $25,000 per year, putting it vastly outside the range of the majority of people who needed it.[82] In 1995, most HIV-positive people in sub-Saharan Africa were living on less than a dollar a day (this has since been raised to about two dollars a day).[83]

Drug-patent laws have been a particular barrier to treatment. Western drug companies took steps to prevent generic drug treatment becoming available because it would violate patent laws,[84] but their own drugs were out of the price range for most of the populations affected by the virus, thus preventing treatment from reaching those who needed it. Some developing countries, such as India and South Africa, decided they would allow violations of patent law for the manufacture of generic antiretrovirals.[85] The drug companies' attempts to sue were only stopped when public outcry in the Western world created bad PR.[86] As a result, middle-income countries are worst affected by the patent problem.[87] The situation is a thorny one: without patents in the first place, the incentive to produce new drugs vanishes. However, the laws as they stand do significant harm to people for the sake of profits.

Furthermore, the drugs were originally not even available in most developing countries. Since imperfect adherence causes the virus to mutate, myths about Africans not understanding time[88] (a myth that was also propagated in an episode of *The West Wing*)[89] contributed to over a decade of delays in the drugs reaching those most in need.[90] Ironically, when the drugs were finally rolled out in 2007, it turned out that Africans were far better than Westerners at taking their medication, thus proving how much these myths were outright wrong.[91]

Former U.S. president Bill Clinton was instrumental in negotiating waivers to costs for some antiretroviral drugs.[92] However, only the initial set of drugs are available for free, with later treatments being held back for salvage therapy when drug resistance inevitably kicks in; no such cost waivers are currently in place for second-line treatment, suggesting a potential humanitarian and economic disaster waiting in the wings.[93]

One of the downsides of lifelong treatment is imperfect adherence to said treatment in the long term, whether due to side effects or pill fatigue.[94] The early drug cocktails had devastating side effects and could often not be used in combination with other medications;[95] lack of cooperation between drug companies meant that patients were often taking up to 26 doses a day, some with food, some without.[96] This led to the need to develop a backup plan for treatment interruptions: short holidays from the drugs, either for medical, lifestyle, or economic reasons.[97]

It was initially thought that interruptions of the order of weeks or months could be tolerated.[98] However, clinical trials that were assessing these breaks had to be halted prematurely as they were killing too many people;[99] instead, mathematical models showed that only short breaks, such as weekends off, could be tolerated.[100]

With the widespread availability of drugs, deaths due to AIDS have plummeted.[101] However, HIV cases continue to rise, as more HIV-positive people are living longer.[102] Indeed, for all the technological development, only two countries have actually reversed their HIV epidemic: Thailand and Uganda.[103] The former used an aggressive condom-awareness campaign that was instigated by the government.[104] The latter accomplished it through traditional medicine.[105] While traditional medicine contains a lot that is scientifically unsound, it has the advantage of tapping into deep societal structures. If the shaman tells you to be faithful, you tend to be faithful.

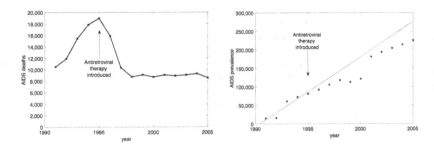

Figure 8.3. *Left:* AIDS deaths among African Americans in the United States, 1990–2005. *Right:* AIDS prevalence among the same group. Note the different scales on the axes. The number of deaths noticeably fell after 1995, while prevalence did not.

Source: R. J. Smith?, 2008.[106]

Unfortunately, significant challenges still remain, in part due to the stigma engendered by the disease's initial assessment. A 2015 outbreak in rural Indiana among injection drug users faced a major obstacle when addicts refused to get tested, fearing that going to a local clinic would have them branded as gay. Many did not know that treatment was available or that sharing used needles was a risk factor.[107]

Other interventions have also been applied to the problem. It was found that circumcised men were less likely to be infected (due to the foreskin retaining vaginal fluid after ejaculation), so a massive circumcision campaign was undertaken.[108] This has the advantage of being a one-time effort and also something that can't be faked.

Vertical transmission (from mother to child) has been almost wholly eliminated, as two doses of nevirapine during childbirth is sufficient to prevent infection.[109] However, babies often get infected later from breast milk.[110] Attempts to circumvent breast milk with technological solutions were not successful;[111] formula requires clean water (which is not always available) and costs money, whereas breast milk is free. Other options were to get the grandmothers to breastfeed, since a simple injection is enough to get any woman to lactate.[112]

However, the real insight was realizing that it was not the breast milk per se that was doing the infecting but rather the breast milk in combination with solid food.[113] A baby's stomach lining is extremely sensitive, and when they first eat solid food, the lining tears, allowing the breast milk to mix with the blood.[114] Instead, there's a much more low-tech solution to the problem of transmission via breast milk: breastfeed initially and then switch to solid food—and never breastfeed again. It's these kinds of solutions, combining scientific insight with cultural sensitivity, that allow us to make progress.

Finally, one of the benefits of the antiretroviral drugs is that they can be used proactively.[115] Medical professionals occasionally have needle-stick incidents, where they accidentally inject themselves with HIV-positive blood.[116] If treatment is started immediately (within about 72 hours of infection), then the virus can be countered before it takes hold.[117] This course of treatment is called post-exposure prophylaxis (PEP)[118] and was for a time being offered directly to the gay community in places such as the annual Gay Pride Festival in Atlanta.[119]

In more recent years, a very different kind of proactive response has emerged: pre-exposure prophylaxis (PrEP). The idea here is for people at risk to take the drugs while they are still HIV-negative, thus preventing infection should they have a risky encounter.[120] PrEP drugs have been termed "chemical condoms," and the prevention rate that they produce is in fact better than condoms if adherence is strong.[121] Innovations such as these illustrate the enormous changes in medical thinking that have been undertaken as a direct response to the AIDS epidemic, which in a very real way has created the global health movement as we know it today.[122] The gay community has thus come full circle, from one that was devastated by this epidemic to one that is proactive and organized, with the prospect of living long and fulfilling lives and enjoying safer condom-free sex, whether HIV-positive or not.

Notes

1. A. Karpas, "Human Retroviruses in Leukaemia and AIDS: Reflections on Their Discovery, Biology and Epidemiology," *Biological Reviews* 79, no. 4 (2004): 911–933.
2. L. K. Altman, "New Homosexual Disorder Worries Health Officials," *The New York Times*, 11 May 1982.
3. W. C. Greene, "A History of AIDS: Looking Back to See Ahead," *European Journal of Immunology* 37, no. S1 (2007): S94–S102.
4. A. Karpas, "Human Retroviruses in Leukaemia and AIDS: Reflections on Their Discovery, Biology and Epidemiology."
5. W. C. Greene, "A History of AIDS: Looking Back to See Ahead."
6. R. C. Gallo, "A Reflection on HIV/AIDS Research after 25 Years," *Retrovirology* 3, no. 1 (2006): 1–7.
7. B. L. Evatt, "The Tragic History of AIDS in the Hemophilia Population, 1982–1984," *Journal of Thrombosis and Haemostasis* 4, no. 11 (2006): 2295–2301.
8. S. Murphy, "Intravenous Drug Use and AIDS: Notes on the Social Economy of Needle Sharing," *Contemporary Drug Problems* 14 (1987): 373–395.
9. C. Butler, "HIV and AIDS, Poverty, and Causation," *The Lancet* 356, no. 9239 (2000): 1445–1446.
10. P. A. Treichler, *How to Have Theory in an Epidemic: Cultural Chronicles of AIDS* (Durham: Duke University Press, 1999).
11. S. S. Karim and G. Ramjee, "Anal Sex and HIV Transmission in Women," *American Journal of Public Health* 88, no. 8 (1998): 1265–1266.
12. P. A. Treichler, *How to Have Theory in an Epidemic: Cultural Chronicles of AIDS*.
13. J. Brier, "Reagan and AIDS," in *A Companion to Ronald Reagan*, ed. A. Johns (Chichester: Wiley Blackwell, 2015), 221–237.
14. A. White, "Reagan's AIDS Legacy: Silence Equals Death," *San Francisco Chronicle*, 8 June 2004.
15. R. Fisher, "The Fiasco of the 1976 'swine flu affair,'" *BBC Future*, 21 September 2020.
16. K. E. Nelson, "Influenza Vaccine and Guillain-Barré Syndrome—Is There a Risk?," *American Journal of Epidemiology* 175, no. 11 (2012): 1129–1132.
17. C. Klein, "When the US Government Tried to Fast-Track a Flu Vaccine," *History. com*, 2 September 2020.

18. P. Mickle, "Fear of a Great Plague," in *The Capital Century, 1900–1999*, ed. J. Blackwell (capitalcentury.com, 1999), 1–7.

19. L. A. Reperant and A. D. Osterhaus, "AIDS, Avian Flu, SARS, MERS, Ebola, Zika... What Next?," *Vaccine* 35 (2017): 4470–4474.

20. M. P. Girard et al., "Human Immunodeficiency Virus (HIV) Immunopathogenesis and Vaccine Development: A Review," *Vaccine* 29 (2011): 6191–6218.

21. B. Lee et al., "Quantification of CD4, CCR5, and CXCR4 Levels on Lymphocyte Subsets, Dendritic Cells, and Differentially Conditioned Monocyte-Derived Macrophages," *Proceedings of the National Academy of Sciences* 96, no. 9 (1999): 5215–5220.

22. E. A. Clark and J. A. Ledbetter, "How B and T Cells Talk to Each Other," *Nature* 367, no. 6462 (1994): 425–428.

23. J. M. den Haan, R. Arens, and M. C. van Zelm, "The Activation of the Adaptive Immune System: Cross-Talk between Antigen-Presenting Cells, T Cells and B Cells," *Immunology Letters* 162, no. 2 (2014): 103–112.

24. J. M. McCune, "The Dynamics of CD4$^+$ T-Cell Depletion in HIV Disease," *Nature* 410, no. 6831 (2001): 974–979.

25. P. W. Nelson, J.E. Mittler, and A. S. Perelson, "Effect of Drug Efficacy and the Eclipse Phase of the Viral Life Cycle on Estimates of HIV Viral Dynamic Parameters," *Journal of Acquired Immune Deficiency Syndromes* 26, no. 5 (2001): 405–412.

26. J. Marshall, "What Does Half-Life Mean?," *Quick and Dirty Tips*, 22 January 2016.

27. P. Lesbats, A. N. Engelman, and P. Cherepanov, "Retroviral DNA Integration," *Chemical Reviews* 116, no. 20 (October 26, 2016): 12730–12757.

28. M. A. Nowak and A. J. McMichael, "How HIV Defeats the Immune System," *Scientific American* 273, no. 2 (1995): 58–65.

29. C. B. Holmes et al., "Review of Human Immunodeficiency Virus Type 1-Related Opportunistic Infections in Sub-Saharan Africa," *Clinical Infectious Diseases* 36, no. 5 (2003): 652–662.

30. M. Woolhouse et al., "Human Viruses: Discovery and Emergence," *Philosophical Transactions of the Royal Society B: Biological Sciences* 367, no. 1604 (2012): 2864–2871.

31. M. A. Nowak and A. J. McMichael, "How HIV Defeats the Immune System."

32. "HIV/AIDS: Snapshots of an Epidemic," *amFAR, the Foundation for AIDS Research,* https://www.amfar.org/thirty-years-of-hiv/aids-snapshots-of-an-epidemic/ (accessed 2 June 2022).

33. J. Cohen, "Reconstructing the Origins of the AIDS Epidemic from Archived HIV Isolates," *Science* 318 (2017): 731.

34. T. Zhu et al., "An African HIV-1 Sequence from 1959 and Implications for the Origin of the Epidemic," *Nature* 391, no. 6667 (1998): 594–597.

35. M. Wayne and B. Bolker, *Infectious Diseases: A Very Short Introduction* (Oxford: Oxford University Press, 2015).

36. J. Pepin, *The Origins of AIDS* (Cambridge: Cambridge University Press, 2021).

37. P. M. Sharp and B. H. Hahn, "Origins of HIV and the AIDS Pandemic," *Cold Spring Harbor Perspectives in Medicine* 1, no. 1 (2011): a006841.

38. F. Van Heuverswyn et al., "SIV Infection in Wild Gorillas," *Nature* 444, no. 7116 (2006): 164.

39. V. M. Hirsch et al., "An African Primate Lentivirus (SIV$_{sm}$) Closely Related to HIV-2," *Nature* 339, no. 6223 (1989): 389–392.

40. P. M. Sharp and B. H. Hahn, "Origins of HIV and the AIDS Pandemic."

41. Z. McMilin, "Knoxville Republican Says AIDS Came from Man Having Sex with a Monkey then with Other Men," *Politifact*, 3 February 2012.

42. M. Peeters et al., "Risk to Human Health from a Plethora of Simian Immunodeficiency Viruses in Primate Bushmeat," *Emerging Infectious Diseases* 8 (2002): 451–457.

43. C. W. McMillen, *Pandemics: A Very Short Introduction* (Oxford: Oxford University Press, 2016).

44. J. Moore. The puzzling origins of AIDS: Although no one explanation has been universally accepted, four rival theories provide some important lesson. *American Scientist* 92, no. 6 (2004): 540–547.

45. C. W. McMillen, *Pandemics: A Very Short Introduction*.

46. "World Bank Says AIDS Threatens South Africa with Economic Collapse," *The New Humanitarian*, 24 July 2003.

47. N. Ansell and L. Young, "Enabling Households to Support Successful Migration of AIDS Orphans in Southern Africa," *AIDS Care* 16, no. 1 (2004): 3–10.

48. J. Witt, "Addressing the Migration of Health Professionals: The Role of Working Conditions and Educational Placements," *BMC Public Health* 9 (2009): S7.

49. P. W. Baur, "Price Setting in the South African Coffin Industry" (master's dissertation, Rand Afrikaans University, 2002).

50. L. Vincent, "Fat in a Time of Slim: The Reinscription of Race in the Framing of Fat Desirability in Post-Apartheid South Africa," *Sexualities* 19, no. 8 (2016): 914–925.

51. C. Tshoose, "The Impact of HIV/AIDS Regarding Informal Social Security: Issues and Perspectives from a South African Context," *Potchefstroom Electronic Law Journal* 13, no. 3 (2010): 407–447.

52. M. Earl-Taylor, "HIV/AIDS, the Stats, the Virgin Cure and Infant Rape," *Science in Africa* (April 2002).

53. C. Hunter-Gault, "Infant Rape Crisis Jolts South Africa," *CNN*, 12 December 2001.

54. S. Bosely, "Mbeki AIDS Policy 'Led to 330,000 Deaths,'" *The Guardian*, 27 November 2008.

55. J. Kitzinger, "The Face of AIDS," in *Representations of Health, Illness and Handicap*, ed. I. Markova and R. Farr (London: Psychology Press, 1995), 49–66.

56. D. Vogl et al., "Symptom Prevalence, Characteristics, and Distress in AIDS Outpatients," *Journal of Pain and Symptom Management* 18, no. 4 (1999): 253–262.

57. J. Esparza, "A Brief History of the Global Effort to Develop a Preventive HIV Vaccine," *Vaccine* 31, no. 35 (2013): 3502–3518.

58. J. Esparza, "An HIV Vaccine: How and When?," *Bulletin of the World Health Organization* 79 (2001): 1133–1137.

59. C. Y. Johnson and L. Bernstein, "Decades of Research on an HIV Vaccine Boost the Bid for One against Coronavirus," *The Washington Post*, 14 July 2020.

60. J. H. Kim, J. L. Excler, and N. L. Michael, "Lessons from the RV144 Thai Phase III HIV-1 Vaccine Trial and the Search for Correlates of Protection," *Annual Review of Medicine* 66 (2015): 423–437.

61. C. P. Batza, "Before AIDS: Gay and Lesbian Community Health Activism in the 1970s" (doctoral dissertation, University of Illinois at Chicago, 2002).

62. N. Aizenman, "How to Demand a Medical Breakthrough: Lessons from the AIDS Fight," *National Public Radio*, 9 February 2019.

63. A. Zuger, "What Did We Learn from AIDS?," *The New York Times*, 11 November 2003.

64. A. Park, "The Story behind the First AIDS Drug," *Time*, 19 March 2017.

65. G. Mousseau, S. Mediouni, and S. T. Valente, "Targeting HIV Transcription: The Quest for a Functional Cure," *Current Topics in Microbiology and Immunology* 389 (2015): 121–145.

66. C. Farber, "AIDS and the AZT Scandal: SPIN's 1989 Feature, 'Sins of Omission,'" *Spin*, 5 October 2015.

67. R. MacArthur, and E. O. Wilson, *The Theory of Island Biogeography* (Princeton: Princeton University Press, 1967).

68. C. Janeway et al., *Immunobiology: The Immune System in Health and Disease*, 6th ed. (New York: Garland Science, 2006).

69. L. Oldach, "Slipping past the Proofreader," *American Society for Biochemistry and Molecular Biology Today*, 10 April 2020.

70. J. D. Roberts, K. Bebenek, and T. A. Kunkel, "The Accuracy of Reverse Transcriptase from HIV-1," *Science* 242, no. 4882 (1998): 1171–1173.

71. G. Pugliese, "Remarkable Discovery Has Implications for HIV Treatment," *Infection Control & Hospital Epidemiology* 16, no. 4 (1995): 250–251.

72. K. Sprouffske et al., "High Mutation Rates Limit Evolutionary Adaptation in *Escherichia coli*," *PLoS Genetics* 14, no. 4 (2018): e1007324.

73. J. M. Kitayimbwa, J. Y. Mugisha, and R. A. Saenz, "Estimation of the HIV-1 Backward Mutation Rate from Transmitted Drug-Resistant Strains," *Theoretical Population Biology* 112 (2016): 33–42.

74. V. Supervie et al., "HIV, Transmitted Drug Resistance, and the Paradox of Preexposure Prophylaxis," *Proceedings of the National Academy of Sciences* 107, no. 27 (2010): 12381–12386.

75. A. Tseng, J. Seet, and E. J. Phillips, "The Evolution of Three Decades of Antiretroviral Therapy: Challenges, Triumphs and the Promise of the Future," *British Journal of Clinical Pharmacology* 79, no. 2 (2015): 182–194.

76. E. J. Arts and D. J. Hazuda, "HIV-1 Antiretroviral Drug Therapy," *Cold Spring Harbor Perspectives in Medicine* 2, no. 4 (2012): a007161.

77. M. M. Zdanowicz, "The Pharmacology of HIV Drug Resistance," *American Journal of Pharmaceutical Education* 70, no. 5 (2006): article 100.

78. B. J. van Welzen, P.G.A. Oomen, and A.I.M. Hoepelman, "Dual Antiretroviral Therapy—All Quiet beneath the Surface?," *Frontiers in Immunology* 12 (2021): article 637910.

79. Z. Lv, Y. Chu, and Y. Wang, "HIV Protease Inhibitors: A Review of Molecular Selectivity and Toxicity," *HIV/AIDS—Research and Palliative Care* 7 (2015): 95–104.

80. J. M. Conway, A. S. Perelson, and J. Z. Li, "Predictions of Time to HIV Viral Rebound following ART Suspension that Incorporate Personal Biomarkers," *PLoS Computational Biology* 15, no. 7 (2019): e1007229.

81. P. L. Vernazza et al., "Potent Antiretroviral Treatment of HIV-Infection Results in Suppression of the Seminal Shedding of HIV," *AIDS* 14, no. 2 (2000): 117–121.

82. N. C. McCann et al., "HIV Antiretroviral Therapy Costs in the United States, 2012–2018," *Journal of the American Medical Association Internal Medicine* 180 (2020): 601–603.

83. M. Ravallion, S. Chen, and P. Sangraula, "Dollar a Day Revisited," *The World Bank Economic Review* 23, no. 2 (2009): 163–184.

84. A. M. Curti, "The WTO Dispute Settlement Understanding: An Unlikely Weapon in the Fight against AIDS," *American Journal of Law & Medicine* 27, no. 4 (2001): 469–485.

85. P. Van Dyck, "Importing Western Style, Exporting Tragedy: Changes in Indian Patent Law and Their Impact on AIDS Treatment in Africa," *Northwestern Journal of Technology and Intellectual Property* 6, no. 1 (2007): 138–151.

86. E. T. Hoen et al., "Driving a Decade of Change: HIV/AIDS, Patents and Access to Medicines for All," *Journal of the International AIDS Society* 14 (2011): 15.

87. O. Mellouk and M. Cassolato, "How Patents Affect Access to HIV Treatment," *Frontline AIDS*, 2 October 2019.

88. V. Dlamini, "What Is this Thing Called African Time?," *Daily Maverick*, 12 January 2020.

89. *The West Wing*, Season 2, Episode 4, "In This White House," 25 October 2000.

90. The United States' war on AIDS. Hearing before the Committee on International Relations, House of Representatives, 107th Congress, 1st session, 7 June 2001, http://commdocs.house.gov/committees/intlrel/hfa72978.000/hfa72978_0.HTM (accessed 2 June 2022).

91. N. C. Ware et al., "Explaining Adherence Success in Sub-Saharan Africa: An Ethnographic Study," *PLoS Medicine* 6, no. 1 (2009): e1000011.

92. M. Liebert, "About AIDS and HIV: A Conversation with President Bill Clinton," *AIDS Patient Care and STDs* 19, no. 9 (2005): xiii–xviii.

93. S. P. Koenig et al., "Monitoring HIV Treatment in Developing Countries," *British Medical Journal* 332 (2006): 602–604.

94. K. G. Buell et al., "Lifelong Antiretroviral Therapy or HIV Cure: The Benefits for the Individual Patient," *AIDS Care* 28, no. 2 (2016): 242–246.

95. C. E. Reust, "Common Adverse Effects of Antiretroviral Therapy for HIV Disease," *American Family Physician* 83, no. 12 (2011): 1443–1451.

96. A. R. Zolopa, "The Evolution of HIV Treatment Guidelines: Current State-of-the-Art of ART," *Antiviral Research* 85 (2010): 241–244.

97. B. M. Adams et al., "Estimation and Prediction with HIV-Treatment Interruption Data," *Bulletin of Mathematical Biology* 69, no. 2 (2007): 563–584.

98. G. Dubrocq and N. Rakhmanina, "Antiretroviral Therapy Interruptions: Impact on HIV Treatment and Transmission," *HIV/AIDS—Research and Palliative Care* 10 (2018): 91–101.

99. B. L. Jewell et al., "Potential Effects of Disruption to HIV Programmes in Sub-Saharan Africa Caused by COVID-19: Results from Multiple Mathematical Models," *The Lancet HIV* 7, no. 9 (2020): e629–e640.

100. A. Turkova et al., "Weekends-off Efavirenz-Based Antiretroviral Therapy in HIV-Infected Children, Adolescents and Young Adults (BREATHER): Extended Follow-up Results of a Randomised, Open-Label, Non-Inferiority Trial," *PLoS ONE* 13, no. 4 (2018): e0196239.

101. S. M. Blower, H. B. Gershengorn, and R. M. Grant, "A Tale of Two Futures: HIV and Antiretroviral Therapy in San Francisco," *Science* 287, no. 5453 (2000): 650–654.

102. F. Nakagawa, M. May, and A. Phillips, "Life Expectancy Living with HIV: Recent Estimates and Future Implications," *Current Opinion in Infectious Diseases* 26 (2013): 17–25.

103. G. Slutkin et al., "How Uganda Reversed Its HIV Epidemic," *AIDS and Behavior* 10, no. 4 (2006): 351–360.

104. W. Rojanapitayakorn, "'100 Percent' Condom Use Seeks to Slow HIV Spread," *Network* 13, no. 4 (1993): 30–32.

105. M. Lamorde et al., "Medicinal Plants Used by Traditional Medicine Practitioners for the Treatment of HIV/AIDS and Related Conditions in Uganda," *Journal of Ethnopharmacology* 130, no. 1 (2010): 43–53.

106. R. J. Smith?, *Modelling Disease Ecology with Mathematics* (American Institute of Mathematical Sciences, 2008).

107. C. W. McMillen, *Pandemics: A Very Short Introduction.*

108. R. Szabo and R. Short, "How Does Male Circumcision Protect against HIV Infection?," *BMJ* 320, no. 7249 (2000): 1592–1594.

109. K. Mukherjee, "Cost-Effectiveness of Childbirth Strategies for Prevention of Mother-to-Child Transmission of HIV among Mothers Receiving Nevirapine in India," *Indian Journal of Community Medicine* 35, no. 1 (2010): 29–33.

110. A. P. Kourtis et al., "Breast Milk and HIV-1: Vector of Transmission or Vehicle of Protection?," *The Lancet Infectious Diseases* 3 (2003): 786–793.

111. G. John-Stewart et al., "Breast-Feeding and Transmission of HIV-1," *Journal of Acquired Immune Deficiency Syndromes* 35 (2004): 196–202.

112. T. A. Ogunlesi et al., "Non-Puerperal Induced Lactation: An Infant Feeding Option in Paediatric HIV/AIDS in Tropical Africa," *Journal of Child Health Care* 12, no. 3 (2008): 241–248.

113. U. Aishat, D. David, and F. Olufunmilayo, "Exclusive Breastfeeding and HIV/AIDS: A Crossectional Survey of Mothers Attending Prevention of Mother-to-Child Transmission of HIV Clinics in Southwestern Nigeria," *Pan African Medical Journal* 21 (2015): article 1.

114. I. Yang et al., "The Infant Microbiome: Implications for Infant Health and Neurocognitive Development," *Nursing Research* 65, no. 1 (2016): 76–88.

115. J. E. Haberer et al., "Real-Time Adherence Monitoring for HIV Antiretroviral Therapy," *AIDS and Behavior* 14, no. 6 (2010): 1340–1346.

116. H. Himmelreich et al., "The Management of Needlestick Injuries," *Deutsches Arzteblatt International* 110, no. 5 (2013): 61–67.

117. N. Angadi, S. Davalgi, and S. S. Vanitha, "Needle Stick Injuries and Awareness towards Post Exposure Prophylaxis for HIV among Private General Practitioners of Davangere City," *International Journal of Community Medicine and Public Health* 3, no. 1 (2016): 335–339.

118. T. N. Young et al., "Antiretroviral Post-Exposure Prophylaxis (PEP) for Occupational HIV Exposure," *Cochrane Database of Systematic Reviews* 1 (2007): article CD002835.

119. S. Kalichman, "Post-Exposure Prophylaxis for HIV Infection in Gay and Bisexual Men: Implications for the Future of HIV Prevention," *American Journal of Preventive Medicine* 15, no. 2 (1998): 120–127.

120. J. E. Volk et al., "No New HIV Infections with Increasing Use of HIV Preexposure Prophylaxis in a Clinical Practice Setting," *Clinical Infectious Diseases* 61, no. 10 (2015): 1601–1603.

121. J. Weber et al., "'Chemical Condoms' for the Prevention of HIV Infection: Evaluation of Novel Agents against $SHIV_{89.6PD}$ in Vitro and in Vivo," *AIDS* 15, no. 12 (2001): 1563–1568.

122. A. M. Brandt, "How AIDS Invented Global Health," *New England Journal of Medicine* 368, no. 23 (2013): 2149–2152.

The Justinianic Plague

In July 541 CE, a disease broke out in the small city of Pelusium at the mouth of the Nile. It travelled the entire Mediterranean basin, reaching as far as Yemen in the South and Finland in the North. It was caused by the bacterium *Yersinia pestis*, which was also responsible for the later bubonic plague in Europe and elsewhere[1] (see chapters 5 and 10) and carried by rats travelling on grain shipments from Egypt to Europe and the Middle East.[2] It also constituted the first historically recorded appearance of true plague.[3]

In Constantinople—which was by that point the capital of the Eastern Roman Empire—people died at such enormous rates that the emperor had to appoint a special officer in charge of coordinating the removal of corpses from the city's streets.[4] It has been estimated that up to 300,000 people died in Constantinople in the first year of the outbreak. Contemporary sources claim that there were approximately 5,000 deaths in the city every day at the height of the pandemic, even reaching 10,000 on some days.[5]

The disease was for many years hypothesized to have come from Africa. Warfare between Byzantium and Persia in the early sixth century had led to close relationships between the Byzantines and Ethiopia's Christian rulers, who were also in close contact with the inhabitants of inner Africa.[6] However, recent genetic evidence suggests an origin in China, travelling along the silk road to Central Asia and to Africa by Chinese marine voyages.[7]

With such an ancient plague, estimates of the precise death toll are unreliable. However, it appears to have killed *between 15 and 100 million*, which accounted for 25%–60% of the Eastern Roman Empire,[8] although some estimates exceed *150 million*.[9] Given the relatively low global population of the time (less than 500 million),[10] this was a substantial blow to the human race. Although this book takes absolute numbers as its metric, it's worth noting that were we to consider proportions of global or regional populations killed, this pandemic would be much higher in the list.

Few named victims exist in the historical records, but one notable person who died from the Justinianic Plague was Pope Pelagius II, who died in 590 CE. Few details of Pelagius's pontificate survive, but his death led to the appointment of his successor, Gregory the Great, whose pontificate coincided with both the end of the plague and a spate of floods.[11]

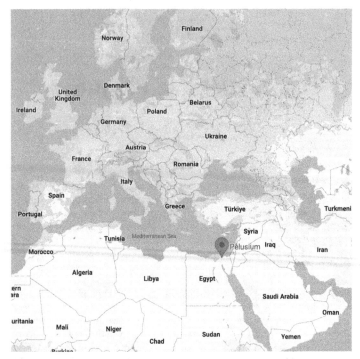

Figure 7.1. Map of the Mediterranean basin, with Finland in the North, the city of Pelusium in the centre, and Yemen in the South, showing the extent of the spread of the Justinianic Plague.

Source: Google Maps.

The disease is named for Emperor Justinian the Great, who reigned over the late Roman Empire from 527–565 CE. Rumours at the time suggested that Justinian created the plague, since emperors were under the direct authority of God;[12] though he didn't create the disease, there's an argument that he did create the pandemic, thanks to the movements of men and bread throughout Justinian's resurrected Empire.[13] Justinian himself was infected but survived, thanks to (or possibly despite) extensive treatment.[14]

Treatment at this time involved cold-water baths, powders "blessed" by saints, magic amulets, and rings, along with various drugs, especially alkaloids. However, those who did survive were credited with good fortune, strong underlying health, and an uncompromised immune system.[15]

As a result of the plague, church taxes were imposed on a pro-rata income basis, which was the forerunner of income taxation. Emperor Justinian increased the tax pressure on his citizens during the plague, in part to pay for countermeasures and in part to pay for ongoing wars. He forced the living to pay not only their own taxes but also those of their dead neighbours.[16] Excessive taxation contributed to the decline of the Eastern Roman Empire and the increasing appeal of Islam, since Muslim conquerors in the wider Empire were perceived by the enslaved inhabitants of the former Roman world as liberators, in particular from excessive taxation.[17] Not only was Islam more tolerant of other religious denominations than Christianity but it also pursued a lenient and pragmatic approach towards taxation: tax rates were moderate, the tax burden was distributed fairly, and tax collection was less corrupt.[18]

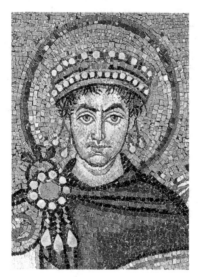

Figure 7.2. Emperor Justinian the Great.
Source: Petar Mološević.

Did the Justinianic Plague contribute to the fall of the Roman Empire? Historians are divided. The minimalist view says no, that nothing major changed, because the mortality patterns were uneven and affected cities much more than all-important agricultural regions.[19] Roman records of administration show continuing economic vitality and no change in land use during the plague period.[20] However, some of the methodology used to determine these factors has been shown to be flawed,[21] and it has been argued that even if the minimalist view is true, the Justinianic Plague's importance as a cultural idea cannot be overstated, because it raised the spectre of how a disease could transform societies.[22]

The historiographical power of the *concept* of a disease is based on three key features: extensive chronology, mortality, and geographic spread.[23] The Justinianic Plague satisfies all three. It transformed religious thinking[24] and was seen as a divine punishment for sins.[25]

The maximalist view says that the plague marked the end of antiquity, the fall of Rome, and the beginning of the Middle Ages.[26] Certainly, such a high death toll has an impact on any society, with a dearth of workers and hence revenue.[27] In fact, the plague was so devastating that it put a significant dent into the world's population growth rate.[28] Part of the lost revenue was in the form of taxation that could pay for the military. The net consequence of this is that the Eastern Roman Empire was left vulnerable to outside attack.

Meanwhile, the lands further to the West had been affected far less by the plague. The urban centres of the Eastern Roman Empire were much more effective breeding grounds for *Y. pestis* than the more rural West; while there were cities there, none of them were on the scale of Constantinople. As such, the Lombards were able to invade, while the Goths took sections of Italy, and the Vandals took Carthage from the Empire's international hold-ings, further reducing Roman income.[29] The Empire had, therefore, not really re-established itself by the time the Ottomans arrived and fought their way to Constantinople, which they captured and held under siege for over a year.[30] The Justinianic Plague could therefore be argued, in the long term, to have contributed to the Eastern Roman Empire's near-defeat at Constantinople in 717 CE.

The Justinianic Plague also had inevitable effects upon the human psyche, with far-reaching consequences. Emperor Justinian saw both the plague and the death of his wife in the mid 540s (CE) as punishments from God.[31] This led to a series of Christian councils held over the next 20 years, during which the divergence between the Eastern Orthodox and Western Catholic churches started.[32] The schism arose from a series of ecclesiastical differences and theological disputes that included whether leavened or unleavened bread should be used in the Eucharist, the celibacy of clerics, the universal juris-diction of the bishop of Rome, and the organization of the church according to Justinianic principles.

The Eastern Roman Empire had been the only great power in Europe. After the Justinianic Plague and the societal changes it wrought, the Empire no longer had military or imperial rule across vast swaths of what had formerly been their land. Without the long arm of Roman control, Europe began to shape itself into the form we recognize today, with the early medi-eval states of the Franks and the Normans (who also took over a chunk of Southern Italy, as well as Normandy and, later, England).[33] Meanwhile, when the Great Schism happened, the Western Catholic Church began to crown its own monarchs, leading to the rise of the Holy Roman Empire.[34]

In short, it can be argued that the Justinianic Plague may have contributed to creating modern Europe as we know it, and it certainly marks the shift from antiquity to the medieval period. The appearance of something so devastating and uncontrollable led to transformative changes in society. As we shall see in the remaining chapters, that will be true of many more modern diseases, not least of which is COVID-19 (though that story is still being written).

The Justinianic Plague was the first. We saw the third in chapter 10. We'll visit the second in a thousand years. But first, we need to take a trip to the twentieth century.

Notes

1. M. Harbeck et al., "*Yersinia pestis* DNA from Skeletal Remains from the 6th Century AD Reveals Insights into Justinianic Plague," *PLoS Pathogens* 9 (2013): e1003349.
2. M. McCormick, "Rats, Communications, and Plague: Toward an Ecological History," *Journal of Interdisciplinary History* 34, no. 1 (2003): 1–25.

3. D. Stathakopoulos, "The Justinianic Plague Revisited," *Byzantine and Modern Greek Studies* 24 (2000): 256–276.

4. C. Wazer, "The Plagues That Might Have Brought Down the Roman Empire," *The Atlantic*, 16 March 2016.

5. A. O'Neill, "Estimates of the Plague of Justinian's Death Toll in Constantinople 541," *Statista*, 8 September 2021.

6. P. Sarris, "The Justinianic Plague: Origins and Effects," *Continuity and Change* 17, no. 2 (2002): 169–182.

7. G. Morelli et al., "Phylogenetic Diversity and Historical Patterns of Pandemic Spread of *Yersinia pestis*," *Nature Genetics* 42, no. 12 (2010): 1140.

8. L. Mordechai et al., "The Justinianic Plague: An Inconsequential Pandemic?," *Proceedings of the National Academy of Sciences* 116 (2019): 25546–25554.

9. A. I. Pogorletskiy and F. Söllner, "Pandemics and Tax Innovations: What Can We Learn from History?," *Journal of Tax Reform* 6, no. 3 (2020): 270–297.

10. C. Haub, "How Many People Have Ever Lived on Earth?," *Population Today* 23, no. 2 (1995): 4–5.

11. L. Mordechai and M. Eisenberg, "Rejecting Catastrophe: The Case of the Justinianic Plague," *Past & Present* 244, no. 1 (2019): 3–50.

12. J. A. S. Evans, *The Age of Justinian: The Circumstances of Imperial Power* (New York: Routledge, 1996).

13. W. Orent, *Plague: The Mysterious Past and Mystifying Future of the World's Most Dangerous Disease* (New York: Free Press, 2004).

14. K. Sessa, "The Justinianic Plague," *Origins: Current Events in Historical Perspective*, 12 June 2020.

15. J. Horgan, "Justinian's Plague (541–542 CE)," *World History Encyclopedia*, 26 December 2014.

16. A. I. Pogorletskiy and F. Söllner, "Pandemics and Tax Innovations: What Can We Learn from History?," *Journal of Tax Reform* 6, no. 3 (2020): 270–297.

17. C. Adams, *For Good and Evil: The Impact of Taxes on the Course of Civilization*, 2nd ed. (Madison: Lanham, 1999).

18. N. A. Lvova and N. V. Pokrovskaya, "Special Features of Islamic Taxation in the Modern Financial System" [in Russian], *Finansy i kredit* 8, no. 632 (2015): 31–40.

19. M. Meier, "The 'Justinianic Plague': The Economic Consequences of the Pandemic in the Eastern Roman Empire and Its Cultural and Religious Effects," *Early Medieval Europe* 24, no. 3 (2016): 267–292.

20. L. Mordechai et al., "The Justinianic Plague: An Inconsequential Pandemic?"

21. P. Sarris, "New Approaches to the 'Plague of Justinian,'" *Past & Present* 254, no. 1 (2021): 315–346.

22. M. Eisenberg and L. Mordechai, "The Justinianic Plague and Global Pandemics: The Making of the Plague Concept," *The American Historical Review* 125, no. 5 (2020): 1632–1667.

23. M. Eisenberg and L. Mordechai, "The Justinianic Plague and Global Pandemics: The Making of the Plague Concept."

24. M. H. Nowak, "The Role of Counterfactual Thinking in the Transformation of Eastern Roman Religiosity towards the Series of Catastrophes of the Justinian Age," *Historyka Studia Metodologiczne* 52 (2022): 327–348.

25. D. Huremović, "Brief History of Pandemics (Pandemics throughout History)," in *Psychiatry of Pandemics: A Mental Health Response to Infection Outbreak*, ed. D. Huremović (Cham: Springer, 2019), 7–35.

26. L. A. White and L. Mordechai, "Modeling the Justinianic Plague: Comparing Hypothesized Transmission Routes," *PLOS One* 15, no. 4 (2020): e0231256.

27. M. Meier, "The 'Justinianic Plague': The Economic Consequences of the Pandemic in the Eastern Roman Empire and Its Cultural and Religious Effects."

28. C. Haub, "How Many People Have Ever Lived on Earth?," *Population Today* 23, no. 2 (1995): 4–5.

29. A. Latham, "Justinian's Plague and the Birth of the Medieval World," https://www.medievalists.net/2020/11/justinian-plague-medieval-world/ (accessed 2 June 2022).

30. T. Zampaki, "The Mediterranean Muslim Navy and the Expeditions Dispatched against Constantinople," *Mediterranean Journal of Social Sciences* 3, no. 10 (2012): 11–20.

31. A. Brown, "Justinian, Procopius, and Deception: Literary Lies, Imperial Politics, and the Archaeology of Sixth-Century Greece," in *Private and Public Lies*, ed. A. Turner, J.K.O. Chong-Gossard, and F. Vervaet (Leiden: Koninklijke Brill NV, 2010), 355–369.

32. R. Hasbrouck, "The First Four Ecumenical Councils as Ineffective Means to Control the Rise and Spread of Heterodox Christian Ideologies," *Undergraduate Research Journal at UCCS* 2, no. 1 (2009): 1–9.

33. I. Shagrir, "Franks and Normans in the Mediterranean: A Comparative Examination of Naming Patterns," *Medieval Prosopography* (2015): 59–72.

34. J. Bryce, *The Holy Roman Empire* (London: Macmillan, 1899).

6 Spanish Flu

I n its first year, COVID-19 killed 1.7 million people and infected more than 50 million, which made it the worst pandemic in more than a century. Recent outbreaks, such as SARS or MERS or Ebola or swine flu, only killed a small fraction of this total, with infections contained geographically.[1] One of the defining features of COVID-19 was its ability to spread globally in a very short space of time.[2] In part, this was because modern transport networks made global travel easily accessible.[3] In 2019, people were moving around the world in vast numbers, creating the perfect conditions for a new disease to quickly spread from an initial outbreak in China to the rest of the world in a matter of months.[4]

A hundred years earlier, another respiratory disease managed to spread around the world for very similar reasons. In 1917, an outbreak of an influenza-like illness was documented at a British military hospital in the Étaples district in France. Clinically, an ordinary case of minor respiratory infection progressed to bronchitis, pneumonia, and then rapidly to death, ushered in by dyspnea and cyanosis.[5] A disease named Spanish flu—later identified as the same one[6]—then arrived in the northern spring of 1918 with a mild wave[7] but roared back with a highly contagious wave in the northern fall of 1918[8] (with a delayed pandemic in the southern hemisphere in between the two).[9] The 2009 swine flu outbreak did much the same thing—which was no surprise, as both were the same influenza strain: H1N1.[10] Prior to 1914, few people travelled long distances, which limited the spread of infectious diseases.[11] However, the First World War changed all that, as troops mobilized back and forth across continents in unprecedented ways.

The average life expectancy in the United States* in 1917 was 51 years.[12] A year later, that had plummeted to 39.[13] This drop was largely due to the Spanish flu.[14] Due to deaths being concentrated in younger individuals (who lacked pre-existing immunity) and women, the birth rate in India had dropped by as much as 30% in 1919.[15] In a single year, this pandemic killed an estimated *50–100 million* people worldwide.[16] That was about 5.5% of the entire world population;[17] this would be equivalent to 430 million deaths today, massively more than COVID-19 or swine flu.

---

* For an extinct or completed cohort (e.g., all people born prior to the 20th century), life expectancy can be calculated by averaging the ages at death. For cohorts with some survivors, it is estimated using mortality experience in recent years.

Indeed, it was worse than the war, which had already taken an enormous global toll, killing 20 million people.[18] The two weren't independent, though; an estimated 40% of the U.S. Navy and 26% of the U.S. Army—more than a million men—became sick with the disease during wartime, with 30,000 dead before they reached the front line.[19] Even the president was not immune: Woodrow Wilson contracted the disease while negotiating the Treaty of Versailles in the immediate aftermath of the war.[20]

Why was Spanish flu so much worse than swine flu, despite being the same influenza strain? Part of the answer is technology: in the intervening 90 years, we've invented ventilators, which can breathe for a patient while the lungs repair themselves.[21] (This is also one of the ways we treat COVID-19 patients.) Part of it is medicine, as antibiotics, which could have treated the worst symptoms of Spanish flu, had not yet been invented. But part of it is also existing immunity: seasonal H1N1 influenza was already circulating when swine flu appeared, which was not the case in 1918.[22] Furthermore, Spanish flu harboured several mutations that were much more virulent than mutations of seasonal H1N1.[23] Finally, a large part of the difference in global impact between the two flus is that general health is simply better a hundred years later.

Deaths from seasonal influenza in each of 1916, 1917, and 1921 were less than a third of the deaths from pandemic influenza in 1918 and 1919.[24] Today, seasonal influenza kills between 300,000 and 700,000 people per year globally,[25] but those numbers have been steadily declining in developed countries for more than a century.[26]

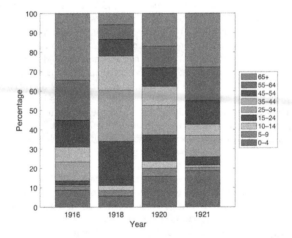

Figure 6.1. Proportional distribution of influenza deaths in Madrid by age. Deaths among young adults increased markedly during 1918.
Source: Created by the author using data from A. Erkoreka, 2010.[27]

The origins of Spanish flu are not precisely known, but one thing is certain: it did not originate in Spain.[28] In fact, it was first seen in an army barracks in Kansas, and subsequent troop movements throughout Europe spread it widely.[29] It may have begun there, or it may have potentially originated in Europe or China.[30]

Troops from rural areas died in much greater numbers than those from urban centres, due to a lack of protective immunity conferred by earlier forms of seasonal influenza.[31] Likewise, isolated places that had not had much contact with the rest of the world suffered large losses; Western Samoa lost 22% of its population to the disease, for example.[32]

The reason the disease became known as Spanish flu is that Spain was not part of the war at the time and hence was not subject to media blackouts.[33] Spain was, therefore, the country that gave the outbreak the most media attention. News of the epidemic was initially suppressed in other countries to avoid damaging morale. Spain's king also contracted the virus, which reinforced the connection.[34]

Diseases have often gone hand-in-hand with wars, due to unsanitary trench conditions, forays into jungles, and mass troop movements.[35] Two thirds of deaths during the American civil war were from dysentery, malaria, typhoid, and pneumonia, while casualties from disease during the Napoleonic wars were eight times that of deaths from battle wounds.[36]

Cultural changes due to the Spanish flu epidemic were significant, but they look familiar in the age of COVID-19.[37] U.S. newspapers printed instructions for people to make their own masks at home, with jail time for those who didn't comply; a special officer in San Francisco even shot a man who refused to wear his.[38] During wartime, mask compliance was high, as it was seen as a way to support the troops, but anti-mask leagues formed after the war.[39] Victims were quarantined, and public spitting was outlawed.[40] There were no nationwide lockdowns,[41] but public theatres, churches, and dance halls were closed down, and library lending was halted.

As the epidemic dragged on, hospitals were overloaded, funeral parlours overwhelmed, and gravediggers in such short supply that people either dug graves for family members or, in northern climates, stored bodies on the roofs of buildings to prevent animal scavenging.[42] In order to go shopping, you'd have to write a list of what you wanted, slip it under the door with some money, and then retreat. The shopkeeper would assemble a package and leave it outside his door. Once he was firmly inside, you'd approach and pick up your goods. Schools were closed for months. In the century between Spanish flu and COVID-19, these may have sounded like extreme or ridiculous measures, but sometimes the old techniques prove useful.

Not everywhere was so cautious. Philadelphia threw a parade to bolster morale and support the war effort, with over 200,000 people jammed into a two-mile stretch, despite the virus having arrived in the city a week prior.[43] Within a week, over 4,500 people had died of the infection,[44] with another 7,500 in the following five weeks.[45] Other responses may sound familiar today: cities such as Tucson and San Francisco were shut down, masks were mandated in public, and students in schools were subject to physical distancing but not masks, as youth were thought to be less susceptible. However, business owners complained about lost revenue, people defied masks or wore them under the nose, and individuals who challenged the mask mandates in court were hailed as champions.[46]

The likelihood of dying from Spanish flu and COVID-19 once you're infected is quite similar. Spanish flu had a case-fatality rate of at least 2.5%, much higher than the 0.1% seen in other influenza pandemics.[47] COVID-19 has an infection-fatality rate of 0.49%–2.53%, although the number increases drastically in older individuals.[48]

The fact that COVID-19 has killed vastly fewer people than Spanish flu is a testament to advances in modern medicine and infrastructure. However, the long-term effects of surviving each of these diseases is quite different: about 4% of Spanish flu survivors suffered ongoing symptoms,[49] compared to 87% of COVID-19 patients.[50]

One of the treatments that was recommended for Spanish flu was aspirin,[51] which had been trademarked in 1899. However, the patent expired in 1917, so new companies were able to produce the drug during the epidemic.[52] Doctors were prescribing doses of up to 30g/day, which is now known to be toxic (doses above 4g/day are considered unsafe).[53] As a result, many people died of aspirin poisoning or suffered symptoms such as hyperventilation, pulmonary edema, or the buildup of fluid in the lungs.[54] Western medicine was no more effective than traditional medicine, leading to strengthened ties to traditional healers; Bombay saw a renewed interest in Ayurvedic and Unani medicine, while Africans associated the taking of European medicine with sickness and death.[55]

High mortality may have also reflected high rates of bacterial infection.[56] Vaccines used during the pandemic were vaccines against a bacterium (*H. influenzae*) that was incorrectly thought to be causing the pandemic.[57] Influenza wasn't known to be a viral disease until the 1930s.[58]

And yet, for all that, Spanish flu was largely forgotten for many decades, barely featuring in most histories of the time or literature.[59] Poor record-keeping and news blackouts reduced the amount of available information, while the deaths were overshadowed by the emotive nature of those from the war, despite being greater in number.[60] For most of the twentieth century, when it was discussed at all, Spanish flu was known as "the forgotten epidemic."[61] That changed in 2009 when H1N1 came back with a vengeance.

The influenza A (H1N1) virus that emerged in April 2009 spread worldwide and generated a pandemic that lasted until August 2010.[62] The virus likely jumped species from influenza in pigs.[63] Symptoms included nasal secretions, chills, fever, and lowered appetite resulting from upper respiratory tract infections.[64] Despite being a subtype of influenza virus A, seasonal flu vaccines offered almost no cross protection against the strain.[65] Whereas typical seasonal influenza epidemics see the vast majority of deaths in individuals aged 65 or older, 80% of those caused by H1N1 were people under 65.[66]

It was at one point suggested that pandemics recur approximately every 90 years, driven in part by the fact that old people were protecting the rest of us: even 90 years on, survivors of Spanish flu still had immunity to the virus, with their blood samples able to neutralize it.[67] However, this theory has been debunked, based on the fact that smaller pandemics have occurred in between these events, caused by different strains of the flu. In the twentieth century, there was also the 1957 Asian flu (flu strain H2N2) and a Hong Kong flu in 1968 (H3N2).[68] In addition, there was a pseudo-pandemic in 1947 with low death rates, a 1977 pandemic in children, and the abortive swine flu epidemic in 1976[69] discussed in chapter 8.

Spanish flu came and went quickly, with the epidemic essentially over in a year,[70] although seasonal flu was unusually high until 1921.[71] There were two waves in the northern hemisphere but only one in the southern hemisphere.[72] Unlike COVID-19, it disappeared quickly because of two factors: mutation to a less transmissible strain, and immunity gained by the survivors.[73]

A direct result of Spanish flu in Canada was the establishment of the Canadian Federal Department of Health, known today as Health Canada, which oversees federal health-related issues, from the Canadian Food Inspection Agency to the Public Health Agency of Canada.[74]

So what lessons did we learn from Spanish flu when it came to COVID-19? On the one hand, very little: most of the major beats of the 1918 pandemic played themselves out a hundred years later. In part, this was because COVID-19 was a very typical pandemic in so many ways. Fortunately, this meant that the usual precautions—masks, distancing, quarantine, vaccination—worked to contain COVID-19,[75] whereas something as complex as HIV/AIDS required a fundamental realignment in thinking. Technology and medical innovation lowered the death toll of COVID-19 relative to Spanish flu, but human behaviour was not drastically different during the two pandemics. It seems that many of the human responses to the COVID-19 pandemic were very much a case of not learning from history and hence being forced to repeat it.

Notes

1. S. Gössling, D. Scott, and C.M. Hall, "Pandemics, Tourism and Global Change: A Rapid Assessment of COVID-19," *Journal of Sustainable Tourism* 29, no. 1 (2020): 1–20.

2. I. Chakraborty and P. Maity, "COVID-19 Outbreak: Migration, Effects on Society, Global Environment and Prevention," *Science of the Total Environment* 728 (2020): 138882.

3. P. Christidis and A. Christodoulou, "The Predictive Capacity of Air Travel Patterns during the Global Spread of the COVID-19 Pandemic: Risk, Uncertainty and Randomness," *International Journal of Environmental Research and Public Health* 17, no. 10 (2020): 3356.

4. C. R. MacIntyre, "Global Spread of COVID-19 and Pandemic Potential," *Global Biosecurity* 1, no. 3 (2020).

5. J. S. Oxford and D. Gill, "A Possible European Origin of the Spanish Influenza and the First Attempts to Reduce Mortality to Combat Superinfecting Bacteria: An Opinion from a Virologist and a Military Historian," *Human Vaccines & Immunotherapeutics* 15, no. 9 (2019): 2009–2012.

6. J. S. Oxford et al., "World War I May Have Allowed the Emergence of 'Spanish' Influenza," *The Lancet Infectious Diseases* 2, no. 2 (2002): 111–114.

7. J. L. Schwartz, "The Spanish Flu, Epidemics, and the Turn to Biomedical Responses," *American Journal of Public Health* 108, no. 11 (2018): 1455–1458.

8. M. Radusin, "The Spanish Flu, Part II: The Second and Third Wave," *Vojnosanitetski Pregled* 69, no. 10 (2012): 917–927.

9. D. M. Morens and A.S. Fauci, "The 1918 Influenza Pandemic: Insights for the 21st Century," *The Journal of Infectious Diseases* 195, no. 7 (2007): 1018–1028.

10. D. Gatherer, "The 2009 H1N1 Influenza Outbreak in Its Historical Context," *Journal of Clinical Virology* 45, no. 3 (2009): 174–178.

11. J. Matthews, "World War One's Role in the Worst Ever Flu Pandemic," *The Conversation*, 5 August 2014.

12. D. W. Smith and B. S. Bradshaw, "Variation in Life Expectancy During the Twentieth Century in the United States," *Demography* 43, no. 4 (2006): 647–657.

13. A. Noymer and M. Garenne, "The 1918 Influenza Epidemic's Effects on Sex Differentials in Mortality in the United States," *Population and Development Review* 26, no. 3 (2000): 565–581.

14. J. K. Taubenberger, "Genetic Characterisation of the 1918 'Spanish' Influenza Virus," in *The Spanish Influenza Pandemic of 1918–1919*, ed. J.S. Oxford, D. Killingray, T. Ranger, and H. Phillips (London: Routledge, 2003), 39–46.

15. C. W. McMillen, *Pandemics: A Very Short Introduction* (Oxford: Oxford University Press, 2016).

16. N. P. Johnson and J. Mueller, "Updating the Accounts: Global Mortality of the 1918–1920 'Spanish' Influenza Pandemic," *Bulletin of the History of Medicine* 1 (2002): 105–115.

17. M. Roser, H. Ritchie, and E. Ortiz-Ospina, "World Population Growth," *Our World in Data*, May 2019, https://ourworldindata.org/world-population-growth (accessed 2 June 2022).

18. P. Wilton, "Spanish Flu Outdid WWI in Number of Lives Claimed," *Canadian Medical Association Journal* 148, no. 11 (1993): 2036.

19. C. R. Byerly, "The US Military and the Influenza Pandemic of 1918–1919," *Public Health Reports* 125, suppl. 3 (2010): 82–91.

20. D. Flecknoe, B. Charles Wakefield, and A. Simmons, "Plagues and Wars: The 'Spanish Flu' Pandemic as a Lesson from History," *Medicine, Conflict and Survival* 34, no. 2 (2018): 61–68.

21. D. M. Morens et al., "The 1918 Influenza Pandemic: Lessons for 2009 and the Future," *Critical Care Medicine* 38, suppl. 4 (2010): e10.

22. W. Kingston, "Antibiotics, Invention and Innovation," *Research Policy* 29, no. 6 (2000): 679–710.

23. G. M. Conenello et al., "A Single Mutation in the PB1-F2 of H5N1 (HK/97) and 1918 Influenza A Viruses Contributes to Increased Virulence," *PLoS Pathogens* 3, no. 10 (2007): e141.

24. A. Erkoreka, "The Spanish Influenza Pandemic in Occidental Europe (1918–1920) and Victim Age," *Influenza and Other Respiratory Viruses* 4, no. 2 (2010): 81–99.

25. A. D. Iuliano et al., "Estimates of Global Seasonal Influenza-Associated Respiratory Mortality: A Modelling Study," *The Lancet* 391, no. 10127 (2018): 1285–1300.

26. P. Doshi, "Trends in Recorded Influenza Mortality: United States, 1900–2004," *American Journal of Public Health* 98, no. 5 (2008): 939–945.

27. A. Erkoreka, "The Spanish Influenza Pandemic in Occidental Europe (1918–1920) and Victim Age."

28. D. Flecknoe, B. Charles Wakefield, and A. Simmons, "Plagues and Wars: The 'Spanish Flu' Pandemic as a Lesson from History."

29. J. M. Barry, "The Site of Origin of the 1918 Influenza Pandemic and Its Public Health Implications," *Journal of Translational Medicine* 2, no. 1 (2004): 1–4.

30. J. S. Oxford, "The So-Called Great Spanish Influenza Pandemic of 1918 May Have Originated in France in 1916," *Philosophical Transactions of the Royal Society of London B: Biological Sciences* 356, no. 1416 (2001): 1857–1859.

31. J. Matthews, "World War One's Role in the Worst Ever Flu Pandemic."

32. S. M. Tomkins, "The Influenza Epidemic of 1918–19 in Western Samoa," *The Journal of Pacific History* 27, no. 2 (1992): 181–197.

33. A. Trilla, G. Trilla, and C. Daer, "The 1918 'Spanish Flu' in Spain," *Clinical Infectious Diseases* 47, no. 5 (2008): 668–673.

34. E. Vázquez-Espinosa, C. Laganà, and F. Vazquez, "The Spanish Flu and the Fiction Literature," *Revista Española de Quimioterapia* 33, no. 5 (2020): 296–312.

35. H. Pennington, "The Impact of Infectious Disease in War Time: A Look Back at WW1," *Future Microbiology* 14, no. 3 (2019): 165–168.

36. M. A. Connolly and D. L. Heymann, "Deadly Comrades: War and Infectious Diseases," *The Lancet* 360 (2002): s23–24.

37. P. M. Munnoli, S. Nabapure, and G. Yeshavanth, "Post-COVID-19 Precautions Based on Lessons Learned from Past Pandemics: A Review," *Journal of Public Health* 4 (2020): 1–9.

38. B. Dolan, "Unmasking History: Who Was behind the Anti-Mask League Protests during the 1918 Influenza Epidemic in San Francisco?," *Perspectives in Medical Humanities* 5, no. 19 (2020).

39. D. K. Nakayama, "Surgical Masks during the Influenza Pandemic of 1918–1920," *The American Surgeon* 86, no. 6 (2020): 557–559.

40. D. Rosner, "'Spanish Flu, or Whatever It Is...': The Paradox of Public Health in a Time of Crisis," *Public Health Reports* 125 (2010): 37–47.

41. A. Sharma et al., "Comparing the Socio-Economic Implications of the 1918 Spanish Flu and the COVID-19 Pandemic in India," *International Social Science Journal* 71, S1 (2021): 23–36.

42. J. Scanlon and T. McMahon, "Dealing with Mass Death in Disasters and Pandemics: Some Key Differences but Many Similarities," *Disaster Prevention and Management* 20, no. 2 (2011): 172–185.

43. M. C. Meinert, "Navigating the 'New Normal' of a Global Pandemic," *American Bankers Association Banking Journal* 112, no. 3 (2020): 30–32.

44. K. C. Davis, "Philadelphia Threw a WWI Parade That Gave Thousands of Onlookers the Flu," *Smithsonian Magazine*, 21 September 2018.

45. L. Asmelash, "Philadelphia Didn't Cancel a Parade during a 1918 Pandemic. The Results Were Devastating," *CNN*, 15 March 2020.

46. B. Luckingham, "To Mask or Not To Mask: A Note on the 1918 Spanish Influenza Epidemic in Tucson," *The Journal of Arizona History* 25, no. 2 (1984): 191–204.

47. J. K. Taubenberger and D. M. Morens, "1918 Influenza: The Mother of All Pandemics," *Revista Biomedica* 17, no. 1 (2006): 69–79.

48. N. F. Brazeau et al., "Estimating the COVID-19 Infection Fatality Ratio Accounting for Seroreversion Using Statistical Modelling," *Communications Medicine* 2 (2022): 54.

49. M. F. Islam, J. Cotler, and L. A. Jason, "Post-Viral Fatigue and COVID-19: Lessons from Past Epidemics," *Biomedicine, Health & Behavior* 8, no. 2 (2020): 61–69.

50. E. Mahase, "COVID-19: What Do We Know about 'Long Covid'?," *British Medical Journal* 370 (2020): m2815.

51. B. Glatthaar-Saalmüller, K. H. Mair, and A. Saalmüller, "Antiviral Activity of Aspirin against RNA Viruses of the Respiratory Tract—An In Vitro Study," *Influenza and Other Respiratory Viruses* 11, no. 1 (2017): 85–92.

52. A. Southerland, "The History of Aspirin: From Willow Bark to Thomas Edison in the 20th Century," *Neurology* 86, no. 16 (2016): P2.391.

53. K. M. Starko, "Salicylates and Pandemic Influenza Mortality, 1918–1919 Pharmacology, Pathology, and Historic Evidence," *Clinical Infectious Diseases* 49, no. 9 (2009): 1405–1410.

54. J. S. Love, A. Blumenberg, and Z. Horowitz, "The Parallel Pandemic: Medical Misinformation and COVID-19," *Journal of General Internal Medicine* 35, no. 8 (2020): 2435–2436.

55. C. W. McMillen, *Pandemics*.

56. J. L. McAuley et al., "Expression of the 1918 Influenza A Virus PB1-F2 Enhances the Pathogenesis of Viral and Secondary Bacterial Pneumonia," *Cell Host & Microbe* 2, no. 4 (2007): 240–249.

57. S. L. Plotkin and S. A. Plotkin, "A Short History of Vaccination," in *Vaccines*, 6th ed., ed. S. Plotkin and W. Orenstein (Philadelphia: Elsevier Saunders, 2013), 1–13.

58. J. K. Taubenberger, "The Origin and Virulence of the 1918 'Spanish' Influenza Virus," *Proceedings of the American Philosophical Society* 150, no. 1 (2006): 86–112.

59. C. W. McMillen, *Pandemics*.

60. L. Martini, "Similarities between Dermal Rashes in Spanish Flu and the 3rd Pandemia of COVID-19," *Our Dematology Online* 12(e) (2021): e57.

61. A. W. Crosby, *America's Forgotten Pandemic: The Influenza of 1918* (Cambridge: Cambridge University Press, 2003).

62. B. A. Sponseller et al., "Influenza A Pandemic (H1N1) 2009 Virus Infection in Domestic Cat," *Emerging Infectious Diseases* 16, no. 3 (2010): 534–537.

63. G. J. Smith et al., "Origins and Evolutionary Genomics of the 2009 Swine-Origin H1N1 Influenza A Epidemic," *Nature* 459, no. 7250 (2009): 1122–1125.

64. S. Echevarría-Zuno et al., "Infection and Death from Influenza A H1N1 Virus in Mexico: A Retrospective Analysis," *The Lancet* 374, no. 9707 (2009): 2072–2079.

65. R. Goodwin et al., "Initial Psychological Responses to Influenza A, H1N1 ('Influenza: Swine Flu')," *BMC Infectious Diseases* 9, no. 1 (2009): 1–6.

66. A. M. Presanis et al., "The Severity of Pandemic H1N1 Influenza in the United States, from April to July 2009: A Bayesian Analysis," *PLoS Medicine* 6, no. 12 (2009): e1000207.

67. E. Yong, "Flu Survivors Still Immune after 90 Years," *National Geographic*, 17 August 2008.

68. P. R. Saunders-Hastings and D. Krewski, "Reviewing the History of Pandemic Influenza: Understanding Patterns of Emergence and Transmission," *Pathogens* 5, no. 4 (2016): 66.

69. E. D. Kilbourne, "Influenza Pandemics of the 20th Century," *Emerging Infectious Diseases* 12, no. 1 (2006): 9–14.

70. H. Markel et al., "Nonpharmaceutical Interventions Implemented by US Cities during the 1918–1919 Influenza Pandemic," *Journal of the American Medical Association* 298, no. 6 (2007): 644–654.

71. A. Erkoreka, "The Spanish Influenza Pandemic in Occidental Europe (1918–1920) and Victim Age."

72. S. Chandra and J. Christensen, "Preparing for Pandemic Influenza: The Global 1918 Influenza Pandemic and the Role of World Historical Information," *Journal of World-Historical Information* 3–4, no. 1 (2016–2017): 19–30.

73. D. Flecknoe, B. Charles Wakefield, and A. Simmons, "Plagues and Wars: The 'Spanish Flu' Pandemic as a Lesson from History."

74. H. Phillips and M. O. Humphries, *The Last Plague: Spanish Influenza and the Politics of Public Health in Canada* (Toronto: University of Toronto Press, 2013).

75. P. P. Bassareo et al., "Learning from the Past in the COVID-19 Era: Rediscovery of Quarantine, Previous Pandemics, Origin of Hospitals and National Healthcare Systems, and Ethics in Medicine," *Postgraduate Medical Journal* 96, no. 1140 (2020): 633–638.

5 The Black Death

Almost a thousand years after the Justinianic Plague arguably led to the fall of the Roman Empire (see chapter 7), plague returned to wreak havoc on Europe.[1] Whereas the Justinianic Plague came and went quickly, inflicting most of its deaths within the first year, the Black Death remained endemic, inflicting damage for more than a century afterwards.[2]

Where do diseases hide between pandemics? It's a complicated question. Some diseases have animal reservoirs, making a zoonotic jump between species[3] (such as H1N1 jumping from pigs to humans in 2009, despite H1N1 having been in humans a century before[4]). Others remain circulating quietly in the off years,[5] infecting people but not on as large a scale as a full-blown pandemic, with particular combinations of loss of immunity and strain mutation leading to a pandemic. Plague has both of these characteristics.[6]

The Black Death was also known as the bubonic plague. The more visceral name is due to the skin turning black shortly before death, due to gangrene.[7] This disease was only recently discovered to have originated in the Chu Valley in Kyrgyzstan in the late 1330s; researchers in 2022 found evidence of the Black Death in skeletons in a Kyrgyzstan graveyard that dated back to the beginning of the bubonic plague, though it's unclear how they were initially infected.[8]

The Black Death swept through Europe in the fourteenth century, killing an estimated *200 million* people.[9] Compare that to the 7–17 million killed by cocoliztli and other haemorrhagic fevers in Mexico over a similar timeframe. Of course, Europe was a lot larger and more populous than Mexico, which gave the Black Death significantly more opportunities to spread and infect.[10] It also infected any number of animals—aside from rats—such as cats, dogs, pigs, and squirrels.[11] So many sheep died during the epidemic that there was a wool shortage across Europe.[12]

Many towns were built like fortresses to keep invaders out, making them ideal for shutting out the infected once the Black Death was underway.[13] Conversely, once the epidemic was inside the walls, it could spread very quickly within an enclosed environment. During the Black Death, villagers learned that it was important to keep strangers out and to isolate and remove anyone infected.[14] This extended to relatives of the infected, possibly out of a belief that it was a curse on the family, but many diseases spread within households, so this likely had a net positive effect.

On the other hand, as the death toll mounted, people began to abandon dying relatives.[15] This led to mass graves being dug in cities, filling with hundreds and sometimes even thousands of bodies.[16] Priests refused to hear confessions, doctors refused to see patients, and shopkeepers closed their doors. The plague was believed to be spread simply by looking at a sick person.[17]

Medieval treatment consisted of animal cures, bloodletting, potions, and fumigations. One of the animal cures involved strapping a plucked chicken to the patient and waiting until the chicken got sick, the thinking being that the disease was being "drawn out" of the patient. Parts of chopped-up snakes were rubbed over the skin, the idea being that evil (of the plague) would be drawn to evil (the snake being synonymous with Satan) and hence leave the body. One of the potions was Four Thieves Vinegar, a combination of cider, vinegar, and wine with spices thought to be a potent protection against the plague. Another potion was theriac, which contained up to 80 ingredients, including significant amounts of opium.[18]

Plague doctors wore beaked masks and all-leather suits in order to provide protection and distance from contamination (though these were not successful). However, their primary responsibility was not to cure or treat the sick but rather administrative: they kept track of the casualties, performed autopsies, and witnessed wills for the dead and dying. Some took advantage of their patients' finances, but they were generally revered, and some were even held for ransom.[19]

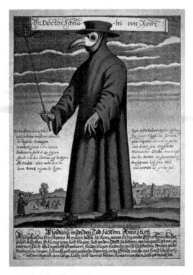

Figure 5.1. Plague doctor's protective outfit.
Source: Wikipedia.

Why did the Black Plague happen when it did, and why did it spread so efficiently across Western Europe? The answer is thought to lie in the 1346 Mongol siege of the village of Kaffa, in Crimea.[20] The Mongols had been moving across Europe, ransacking and pillaging as they went. However, Kaffa was ready for them: it was a walled city on a port, with a river flowing through it.[21] Residents had stocked up and had experience of sieges, so they hunkered down with enough supplies of food and water to outlast the Mongols. Faced with this impasse, the Mongols did what anyone would do: they invented a bioweapon.[22]

There were plenty of dead bodies around, so the Mongols catapulted some of them over the walls, intending to "smoke out" the villagers.[23] The bodies rotted, and the plague spread in earnest. Faced with threats from the inside and the outside, many residents fled by sea,[24] taking ships to Constantinople, one of the biggest metropolitan centres of the time. And they took the plague with them.[25]

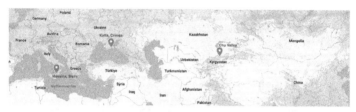

Figure 5.2. Map of Europe showing Messina (east), Kaffa (centre), and Chu Valley (west). *Source:* Google Maps.

When ships arrived in Messina, Sicily, in 1347, residents were shocked to discover that most onboard were dead, and those who weren't were infected.[26] The "ships of the dead" were ordered to leave, but it was too late; the pandemic had already begun to spread.[27] Ships were particularly efficient carriers of the disease, because the rats that harboured the infected fleas flourished in the holds, feeding on grain and other supplies.[28]

Superstition was rife, with many people blaming witches for the plague's devastation.[29] Since cats were the familiars of witches, people began killing cats;[30] unfortunately, this removed one of the rats' major urban predators, allowing the disease to spread even further.[31] (Although cats can carry and transmit plague themselves,[32] in areas where cats were numerous, no plague occurred.[33]) There are parallels here to the role of social media and anti-vaccine propaganda in COVID-19, with the very things that could solve the epidemic under attack when we listen to hearsay rather than fact.[34]

Witches weren't the only ones thought to be responsible; people believed that the local Jews had poisoned the wells and thus began large-scale persecution and execution,[35] entirely eliminating Jewish areas from cities such as Mainz and Cologne.[36] Many Jews fled to Poland, where they were welcomed and remained until the Second World War.[37]

The Mongols themselves got infected but continued their ransacking of Europe, taking the plague with them. As a result, the Black Death had multiple sources, like a fire catching in several places at once.[38] The spread of the disease was incredible for a pre-industrial era: at its peak, the Black Death travelled across Europe at a rate of five kilometres per day, which is incredibly fast for a disease.[39] By comparison, the 1899–1925 plague in South Africa spread no faster than 8 to 12 miles per *year*.[40]

Faced with such an overwhelming situation, many people believed they were being punished by God and living in the end times.[41] The church at the time was immensely powerful, but any advice that priests gave was ineffective against the disease. Priests themselves started dying, which caused people to lose faith and broke the back of the church's power, with the faithful turning to other forms of spirituality.[42]

The flagellant movement was one. Some people had believed that public displays of self-flagellation (whipping one's own back with leather straps studded with metal) would be appropriate penance in God's eyes.[43] During the plague, upper-class men joined this movement, marching through cities. So popular was this that it threatened the authority of the pope, who shut it down.[44]

The church wasn't the only entity to lose power in the face of the Black Death.[45] The power dynamics of fiefdoms and city states crumpled, as workers died and people fled cities. In fact, so many serfs died that there was a significant labour shortage. There was thus a need to find labour elsewhere, which led to colonization, in order to open trade and find slaves who could replace the missing workers.[46]

The plague killed the 13-year-old son of the Byzantine emperor when plague-laden ships docked in Constantinople, but he wasn't alone.[47] During the first five years of the Black Death, 20 million Europeans died, about a third of the continent.[48] Proportionally speaking, this made it the most fatal single pandemic in history.[49] In 1542, it may have killed Lisa del Giocondo, an Italian noblewoman from an aristocratic family, otherwise known as the Mona Lisa,[50] several decades after she sat for da Vinci.[51] All told, the Black Death persisted for around 400 years, with Marseilles experiencing a massive epidemic in the 1720s and a final outbreak in Moscow in 1770.[52]

The Black Death has been instrumental in shaping much of Western civilization due to its impact on the development of European societies, even centuries later. Most importantly, it was during the circumstances surrounding this disease that quarantine was developed. In 1377, a 30-day holding period for incoming ships (known in Italian as a *trentino*) was introduced in the city of Ragusa, Croatia;[53] it was later increased to 40 days (*quarantino*),[54] possibly chosen because the number 40 had biblical significance, with the Great Flood of 40 days and 40 nights or Jesus fasting in the wilderness for 40 days. This had the desired effect of slowing the disease down. The invention of quarantine is regarded as one of the high points of medieval medicine.[55]

Quarantine is still an enormously effective method of disease control, and not just for humans. Animals are more easily quarantined than obstinate humans, and animal husbandry often involves a series of disconnected barns or fields so that diseases can be easily contained if an outbreak occurs.[56] For example, the cow and buffalo disease rinderpest, also known as "cattle plague" (though unrelated to the bubonic plague; it's closely related to measles),[57] was successfully controlled and eliminated from Europe in the 1990s using quarantine and hygienic measures.[58]

The Black Death had other effects on our current habits. It killed off many of the monks who were trained to painstakingly copy religious texts, which—along with the availability of cheap paper—led to the invention of the printing press,[59] which in turn made books much more accessible to the public, increasing literacy exponentially.[60] Survivors inherited land, and food prices dropped significantly, as did land values, which led to the end of feudalism.[61] Culturally, the Black Death led to the Renaissance, as the plague had thinkers dwelling more on life on Earth than spirituality and the afterlife, which moved art and literature away from its religious focus and more towards a secular understanding of humanity.[62] The reason we bury bodies six feet under is because that was the depth that was thought to protect people from infection by corpse.[63] You can imagine the trial and error that led to this determination.

Under immense pressure, traits that might otherwise not be so successful can be selected by evolution.[64] During the Black Death, a few people had a random mutation where they were missing a receptor on their T cells.[65] This would not normally be beneficial, as these receptors help the immune system communicate information about new infections. However, without this receptor, the bacterium was unable to infect the T cells. This made those people immune to the infection. With so many deaths, anyone with an advantage is more likely to breed and pass on those mutations to their descendants.[66] This is exactly what happened.

Today, about 10% of the European population is missing that receptor. What's amazing is that this makes them immune to HIV, since that virus also cannot attach to the T cells.[67] (See chapter 8.) This property was used to design one class of HIV drugs, called entry inhibitors, which served to block viral entry at the receptor for the rest of us who still have it.[68] What's tragic is that HIV is an enormous problem in Africa, because their ancestors, having escaped the Black Death in the fifteenth century, means Africans today have almost no natural immunity to HIV.[69]

This missing T-cell receptor wasn't the only trait selected for by evolution as a result of the Black Plague. Recent evidence showed that various auto-immune disorders we know today, such as rheumatoid arthritis and Crohn's disease, are linked to a gene variant that was selected for by the plague. This variant, known as ERAP 2, was present in 40% of Londoners before the Black Death, rising to 50% afterwards. However, in some parts of the world, the disparity was much greater, rising from 45% to 70% in Denmark.[70] It's unknown whether this variant confers protection against other pathogens.

Bubonic plague isn't gone, but since 1928 it can be treated with antibiotics,[71] as mentioned in chapter 10. Following the introduction of antibiotics, the case-fatality rate is now down to 11%, which is better than it was, but the plague still kills 3,000 people each year.[72]

The bacterium that causes the plague has barely shifted in 700 years: DNA from skeletons in fourteenth-century London shows an almost identical plague to the outbreak in Madagascar in 2013.[73] This was just one of several post–Third Plague outbreaks: a 1994 outbreak in the city of Surat, India, led to media reports of plague in that province, which in turn caused people to flee the province, thus taking the plague with them across the country.[74]

About 300,000 people fled Surat in two days, the largest post-independence migration of people in India.

The media's relationship with diseases in a complex one, and the 1994 outbreak of plague in India is an excellent case study. Media outlets thrive on sensationalism, especially when focused on a few cases that can have a human-interest angle. This makes the media very effective at the beginning of a pandemic but less interested after one is underway. As seen in the 1994 Indian outbreak, media influences behaviour, but behaviour also influences media (subsequent reports detailed the spreading of the plague across India with no acknowledgement of the media's role in precipitating the spread).[75]

Despite the plague bacterium's DNA stability across centuries, another threat looms: the possibility of drug resistance.[76] The bubonic plague is well-controlled by antibiotics, but other diseases such as gonorrhea have developed such efficient resistance that they are effectively uncontrollable now.[77] This isn't just a hypothetical fear; antibiotic-resistant strains of the plague were seen in Madagascar in 1995. Resistance to antibiotics is not just a matter of human use; humans didn't invent antibiotics but rather co-opted them from fungi, so antibiotic-resistant genes have been extracted from 30,000-year-old frozen soil.[78] Should the plague further mutate in this way, we could be facing a resurgent pandemic of terrifying proportions.[79]

Notes

1. L. Mordechai et al., "The Justinianic Plague: An Inconsequential Pandemic?," *Proceedings of the National Academy of Sciences* 116, no. 51 (2019): 25546–25554.
2. L. Wade, "From Black Death to Fatal Flu, Past Pandemics Show Why People on the Margins Suffer Most," *Science*, 14 May 2020.
3. R. Rosenberg, "Detecting the Emergence of Novel, Zoonotic Viruses Pathogenic to Humans," *Cellular and Molecular Life Sciences* 72, no. 6 (2015): 1115–1125.
4. M. L. Flanagan et al., "Anticipating the Species Jump: Surveillance for Emerging Viral Threats," *Zoonoses and Public Health* 59, no. 3 (2012): 155–163.
5. U. Khan et al., "Pandemics of the Past: A Narrative Review," *The Journal of the Pakistan Medical Association* 70, no. 5 (2020): S34–S37.
6. A. Bramanti et al., "Plague: A Disease which Changed the Path of Human Civilization," in *Yersinia pestis: Retrospective and Perspective*, ed. R. Yang and A. Anisimov (Dordrecht: Springer Nature BV, 2016), 1–26.
7. K. A. Glatter and P. Finkelman, "History of the Plague: An Ancient Pandemic for the Age of COVID-19," *The American Journal of Medicine* 134, no. 2 (2021): 176–181.
8. I. Sample, "Mystery of Black Death's Origins Solved, Say Researchers," *The Guardian*, 15 June 2022.
9. K. Philipkoski, "Black Death's Gene Code Cracked," *Wired*, 3 October 2001.
10. R. Acuña-Soto et al., "Megadrought and Megadeath in 16th Century Mexico," *Emerging Infectious Diseases* 8 (2002): 360–362.
11. A. Bramanti et al., "Plague: A Disease which Changed the Path of Human Civilization."
12. W. M. Bowsky, "The Impact of the Black Death upon Sienese Government and Society," *Speculum* 39, no. 1 (1964): 1–34.
13. P. Slack, "The Black Death Past and Present. 2. Some Historical Problems," *Transactions of the Royal Society of Tropical Medicine and Hygiene* 83, no. 4 (1989): 461–463.

14. P. Slack, "Responses to Plague in Early Modern Europe: The Implications of Public Health," *Social Research* 55, no. 3 (1988): 433–453.

15. D. Herlihy and S. H. Cohn, *The Black Death and the Transformation of the West* (Boston: Harvard University Press, 1997).

16. M. A. Spyrou et al., "Historical *Y. pestis* Genomes Reveal the European Black Death as the Source of Ancient and Modern Plague Pandemics," *Cell Host & Microbe* 19, no. 6 (2016): 874–881.

17. R. Hajar, "The Air of History (Part II) Medicine in the Middle Ages," *Heart Views* 13, no. 4 (2012): 158–162.

18. J. J. Mark, "Medieval Cures for the Black Death," *World History Encyclopedia*, 15 April 2020.

19. D. Rennie, "Inside the Terrifying but Necessary Job of a Medieval Plague Doctor," *All That's Interesting*, 16 August 2022.

20. H. Ditrich, "The Transmission of the Black Death to Western Europe: A Critical Review of the Existing Evidence," *Mediterranean Historical Review* 32, no. 1 (2017): 25–39.

21. P. Shipman, "The Bright Side of the Black Death," *American Scientist* 102, no. 6 (2014): 410–413.

22. M. K. McLendon, M. A. Apicella, and L. A. Allen, "*Francisella tularensis*: Taxonomy, Genetics, and Immunopathogenesis of a Potential Agent of Biowarfare," *Annual Reviews of Microbiology* 60 (2006): 167–185.

23. F. Frischknecht, "The History of Biological Warfare: Human Experimentation, Modern Nightmares and Lone Madmen in the Twentieth Century," *EMBO reports* 4, S1 (2003): S47–S52.

24. C. McEvedy, "The Bubonic Plague," *Scientific American* 258, no. 2 (1988): 118–123.

25. M. Wheelis, "Biological Warfare at the 1346 Siege of Caffa," *Emerging Infectious Diseases* 8, no. 9 (2002): 971–975.

26. E. Tognotti, "Lessons from the History of Quarantine, from Plague to Influenza A," *Emerging Infectious Diseases* 19, no. 2 (2013): 254–259.

27. R. Hajar, "The Air of History (Part II) Medicine in the Middle Ages."

28. B. Bramanti et al., "The Third Plague Pandemic in Europe," *Proceedings of the Royal Society B* 286, no. 1901 (2019): 20182429.

29. A. M. Schultz, "Maleficium and Witchcraft: How Being a Witch and Magic Was Viewed in Early Modern Europe," *Exemplore*, 2 July 2020.

30. C. I. Cox, "Plague like Cats: Soft Instruments of Sharp Justice in William Baldwin's Beware the Cat," *Explorations in Renaissance Culture* 41, no. 1 (2015): 1–29.

31. E. A. Lawrence, "Feline Fortunes: Contrasting Views of Cats in Popular Culture," *Journal of Popular Culture* 36, no. 3 (2003): 623–635.

32. C. A. Ross, *Fear and Disease: Black Plague and Cultural Interactions throughout Recorded History* (Fullerton: California State University, 1995).

33. A. Buchanan, "Enquiries Regarding the Mode of Spread and the Prevention of Plague," *The Indian Medical Gazette* 43, no. 8 (1908): 292–294.

34. N. Puri et al., "Social Media and Vaccine Hesitancy: New Updates for the Era of COVID-19 and Globalized Infectious Diseases," *Human Vaccines & Immunotherapeutics* 16, no. 11 (2020): 2586–2593.

35. T. Finley and M. Koyama, "Plague, Politics, and Pogroms: The Black Death, the Rule of Law, and the Persecution of Jews in the Holy Roman Empire," *The Journal of Law and Economics* 61, no. 2 (2018): 253–277.

36. S. K. Cohn, "The Black Death and the Burning of Jews," *Past and Present* 196, no. 1 (2007): 3–6.

37. J. van Straten, "Jewish Migrations from Germany to Poland: the Rhineland Hypothesis Revisited," *Mankind Quarterly* 44, no. 3–4 (2003): 367–384.

38. M. H. Green, "The Four Black Deaths," *The American Historical Review* 125, no. 5 (2020): 1601–1631.

39. S. K. Cohn, "Epidemiology of the Black Death and Successive Waves of Plague," *Medical History* 52, S27 (2008): 74–100.

40. G. Twigg, *The Black Death: A Biological Reappraisal* (New York: Schocken Books, 1985).

41. A. Foa, *The Jews of Europe after the Black Death* (Berkeley: University of California Press, 2000).

42. W. J. Dohar, *The Black Death and Pastoral Leadership* (Philadelphia: University of Pennsylvania Press, 2018).

43. R. Kieckhefer, "Radical Tendencies in the Flagellant Movement of the Mid-Fourteenth Century," *Journal of Medieval and Renaissance Studies* 4, no. 2 (1974): 157–176.

44. M. H. Zentner, "The Black Death and Its Impact on the Church and Popular Religion" (honour's thesis, University of Mississippi, 2015).

45. R. Jedwab, N. Johnson, and M. Koyama, "The Economic Impact of the Black Death," *Journal of Economic Literature* 60, no. 1 (2022): 132–178.

46. E. D. Domar, "The Causes of Slavery or Serfdom: A Hypothesis," *Journal of Economic History* 30, no. 1 (1970): 18–32.

47. C. S. Bartsocas, "Two Fourteenth Century Greek Descriptions of the 'Black Death,'" *Journal of the History of Medicine and Allied Sciences* 21, no. 4 (1966): 394–400.

48. A. L. DesOrmeaux, "The Black Death and Its Effect on Fourteenth- and Fifteenth-Century Art" (master's thesis, Louisiana State University and Agricultural and Mechanical College, 2007).

49. D. W. Gingerich and J. P. Vogler, "Pandemics and Political Development: The Electoral Legacy of the Black Death in Germany," *World Politics* 73, no. 3 (2021): 393–440.

50. C. Kucharz, "Revealed: The Identity of Leonardo's 'Mona Lisa,'" *ABC News*, 17 January 2008.

51. B. Davis, "How Did the Mona Lisa Impact Society?," *MVOrganizing*, 9 August 2019.

52. P. Slack, "Perceptions of Plague in Eighteenth-Century Europe," *The Economic History Review* 75, no. 1 (2022): 138–156.

53. P. A. Mackowiak and P. S. Sehdev, "The Origin of Quarantine," *Clinical Infectious Diseases* 35, no. 9 (2002): 1071–1072.

54. T. Chorba, "Social Distancing and Artful Pandemic Survival," *Emerging Infectious Diseases* 26, no. 11 (2020): 2793–2794.

55. A. A. Conti, "Quarantine through History," *International Encyclopedia of Public Health* (2008): 454–461.

56. K. Brown and D. Gilfoyle, *Healing the Herds: Disease, Livestock Economies, and the Globalization of Veterinary Medicine* (Athens: Ohio University Press, 2010).

57. M. Wayne and B. Bolker, *Infectious Diseases: A Very Short Introduction* (Oxford: Oxford University Press, 2015).

58. T. Barrett and P. B. Rossiter, "Rinderpest: The Disease and Its Impact on Humans and Animals," *Advances in Virus Research* 53 (1999): 89–110.

59. C. Adams, "Did You Know...Fascinating Printing Facts," *Printing Impressions*, 1 February 2015.

60. E. L. Eisenstein, *The Printing Press as an Agent of Change* (Cambridge: Cambridge University Press, 1980).

61. W. Scheidel, *The Great Leveler* (Princeton: Princeton University Press, 2017).

62. J. E. Jost, "The Effects of the Black Death: The Plague in Fourteenth-Century Religion, Literature, and Art" in *Death in the Middle Ages and Early Modern Times*, ed. A. Classen (Berlin: de Gruyter, 2016), 193–238.

63. D. Defoe, *A Journal of the Plague Year* (London: E. Nutt, 1722).

64. A. Sih, M. C. Ferrari, and D. J. Harris, "Evolution and Behavioural Responses to Human-Induced Rapid Environmental Change," *Evolutionary Applications* 4, no. 2 (2011): 367–387.

65. C. J. Duncan and S. Scott, "What Caused the Black Death?," *Postgraduate Medical Journal* 81, no. 955 (2005): 315–320.

66. P. C. Sabeti et al., "The Case for Selection at CCR5-Δ32," *PLoS Biology* 3, no. 11 (2005): e378.

67. S. R. Duncan, S. Scott, and C. J. Duncan, "Reappraisal of the Historical Selective Pressures for the CCR5-Δ32 Mutation," *Journal of Medical Genetics* 42, no. 3 (2005): 205–208.

68. J. P. Moore and R. W. Doms, "The Entry of Entry Inhibitors: A Fusion of Science and Medicine," *Proceedings of the National Academy of Science* 100 (2003): 10598–10602.

69. J. C. Stephens et al., "Dating the Origin of the CCR5-Δ32 AIDS-Resistance Allele by the Coalescence of Haplotypes," *The American Journal of Human Genetics* 62, no. 6 (1998): 1507–1515.

70. K. Hunt, "The Black Death Is Still Affecting the Human Immune System," *CNN*, 19 October 2022.

71. W. R. Byrne et al., "Antibiotic Treatment of Experimental Pneumonic Plague in Mice," *Antimicrobial Agents and Chemotherapy* 42, no. 3 (1998): 675–681.

72. T. Butler, "The Black Death Past and Present. 1. Plague in the 1980s," *Transactions of the Royal Society of Tropical Medicine and Hygiene* 83, no. 4 (1989): 458–460.

73. A. Lawler, "How Europe Exported the Black Death," *Science*, 29 April 2016.

74. V. Ramalingaswami, "Psychosocial Effects of the 1994 Plague Outbreak in Surat, India," *Military Medicine* 166 (2001): 29–30.

75. J. M. Tchuenche et al., "The Impact of Media Coverage on the Transmission Dynamics of Human Influenza," *BMC Public Health* 11, suppl. 1 (2011): S5.

76. N. C. Stenseth et al., "Plague: Past, Present, and Future," *PLoS Medicine* 5, no. 1 (2008): e3.

77. A. R. Tuite et al., "Impact of Rapid Susceptibility Testing and Antibiotic Selection Strategy on the Emergence and Spread of Antibiotic Resistance in Gonorrhea," *The Journal of Infectious Diseases* 216, no. 9 (2017): 1141–1149.

78. M. Wayne and B. Bolker, *Infectious Diseases: A Very Short Introduction*.

79. B. J. Hinnebusch, "High-Frequency Conjugative Transfer of Antibiotic Resistance Genes to *Yersinia pestis* in the Flea Midgut," *Molecular Microbiology* 46, no. 2 (2002): 349–354.

4 Measles

O ften written off as a harmless childhood disease, measles' appearance in the top ten might seem surprising to anyone born after the
invention of the internet. Infection is extremely common, as its high
transmissibility used to mean that pretty much all children became
infected, and most recovered.[1] Indeed, since the risk of severe side effects is
higher later in life, parents would often host "measles parties" for kids, in
order to get the infection out of the way as quickly as possible.[2]

Symptoms range from the mild to the wild, with common symptoms
being a telltale red rash, fever, and flu-like symptoms, as well as Koplik's
spots in the mouth; these are white dots that are temporary but are used
to diagnose measles.[3] However, complications are also common, including
diarrhoea, pneumonia, brain inflammation, and corneal scarring.[4]

Measles evolved from rinderpest, jumping from cattle to humans in the
sixth century.[5] Rinderpest is one of only two diseases we've eradicated,
thanks to a successful vaccine, and its symptoms are quite different from
measles: they include fever, oral erosions, diarrhoea, lymphoid necrosis, and
high mortality.[6] Rinderpest was likely responsible for the emergence of an
entirely different disease: it wiped out the native wildlife in East Africa,
which allowed the growth of shrubby vegetation, a natural habitat for tsetse
flies, which in turn allowed sleeping sickness to become established.[7]

Although the majority of infectious diseases in humans emerged after
the Neolithic revolution, it's thought that measles' much later emergence
may have coincided with the rise of large cities; populations large enough
to support continuous measles transmission could not exist in Neolithic,
Bronze Age, and early Iron Age settlements, which lacked both economic
and political means to support such numbers.[8] The reason diseases started
accelerating with the advent of modern farming practices was because we
were living much closer to animals.[9]

The first written record of measles dates back to ninth century Persia,
when a physician named Rhazes of Baghdad differentiated it from smallpox.[10]
Its viral pathogen was identified in 1757 by Francis Home, a Scottish doctor
who first attempted to make a vaccine. Measles has killed *200 million* people
in the past 165 years alone (dating back to 1855).[11] Mostly these were children
under five in developing countries.

There's no treatment for measles itself, but treatments exist for some
of its symptoms.[12] Antibiotics can help, even though antibiotics don't work

against viruses, because some of the symptoms are bacterial.[13] If you catch measles and survive, symptomatic immunity is essentially lifelong; asymptomatic infection can sometimes occur, but reappearance of symptoms is extremely rare.[14]

Although most people survive the infection, the reason for its high death toll is that it's highly transmissible, so the chances of an adverse reaction simply go up.[15] As we all now know thanks to COVID-19,* the reproduction number, R_0, measures the average number of secondary infections that an infected person creates in a wholly susceptible population during their infectious lifetime.[16] It's essentially a measure of infection speed; if R_0 is larger than 1, then each infected individual is creating, on average, more infected individuals than themselves. An R_0 of 3 means that the first infected individual infects three people, who each infect three more, making nine, then 27, 81, and so forth.[17] In reality, it doesn't always continue to grow like this because we run out of susceptibles; some of those 81 people might already be infected or immune, so the transmission gets "wasted" on them.

Conversely, if R_0 is less than 1, then each infected person is leaving behind fewer infected people than themselves. Ten people might infect nine, nine infect eight, and so on until the disease disappears, though the final outcome is highly dependent on chance effects.[18] Knowing R_0 gives us a way of understanding a disease's prevalence. Even better, it tells us when our intervention methods will be sufficient, because if we quarantine, vaccinate, and treat enough people to flip the R_0 below 1, then the disease will stop expanding and start shrinking.[19]

Most diseases have an R_0 somewhere around 1.5–2. COVID-19, which is famous for its high transmissibility, had an initial R_0 of 2.5. (We've since brought that down, thanks to masks, social distancing, and vaccination,[20] although later variants have much higher reproduction numbers.)[21] However, measles has an R_0 of 17, which is staggeringly high.[22] This means that if a single child with measles arrives at a school where no one has any immunity, she'll infect 17 classmates, each of whom will go on to infect many more, and before long the entire school is awash with measles.[23] The omicron variant of COVID-19 has a reproduction number of 9.5, although the range goes up to 24.[24] Stopping these diseases is very challenging.

Of course, this doesn't actually happen in schools these days, because of pre-existing immunity thanks to earlier measles infections or vaccination (it would be rare to find a school made up of entirely susceptible children). However, that wasn't the case for some parts of the world: island nations, for example, with no pre-existing immunity.[25] In 1529, a measles outbreak in Cuba killed two thirds of the indigenous population.[26] In 1531, fully half the population of Honduras died of it.[27] An 1875 outbreak in Fiji wiped out a third of the population in four months,[28] and a third of Hawaiians also died from it in 1848. Hawaii's king and queen contracted it and died in 1824 while taking an overseas trip.[29] Measles has a tendency to sweep through populations, either killing them or providing the survivors with immunity.

---

* Or possibly from the 2011 movie *Contagion,* one of the better Hollywood portrayals of a pandemic.

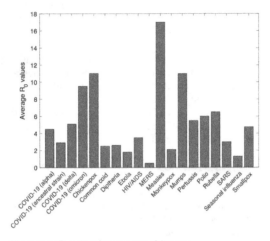

Figure 4.1. R_0 values for a variety of diseases.
Source: Created by the author using data from Wikipedia.

When he was 12, Mark Twain deliberately exposed himself to a friend with measles and almost died as a result.[30] Some NCAA basketball teams played multiple games during the 1988–1989 seasons to empty stadiums due to an outbreak of measles.[31] Children's author Roald Dahl lost his seven-year-old daughter to measles encephalitis in 1962. (He dedicated *The Big Friendly Giant* to her memory.)[32] Just a year later, a safe and effective vaccine became available.

A vaccine had originally been developed in 1954 by John Enders, but it was quite toxic.[33] Children who received the vaccine often had fevers so high that they had seizures.[34] In 1963, the vaccine was refined by Maurice Hilleman, who created a safe and highly effective measles vaccine that is still used today.[35] (Roald Dahl became a pro-vaccination advocate.)

Hilleman is one of the unsung heroes of the twentieth century. He and his lab were responsible for developing vaccines against measles, mumps, hepatitis A, hepatitis B, meningitis, pneumonia, influenza, and rubella.[36] This is a remarkable 8 out of 14 vaccines routinely recommended in developed countries today. Indeed, Hilleman is responsible for developing more vaccines than any other person in history.[37]

In 1963, when Hilleman's daughter had mumps, he swabbed the back of her throat, brought it to the lab, and by 1967 had developed a mumps vaccine,[38] with her baby sister one of the first to receive the experimental vaccine.[39] Although a firebrand of a personality—he had exacting standards and kept fake shrunken heads in his office for every employee he'd fired—Hilleman did not seek fame or recognition for his work and is thus largely unknown today.[40] His vaccines are estimated to save eight million lives each year.[41]

In fact, several of Hilleman's vaccines are nowadays combined into a single shot. The measles–mumps–rubella (MMR) combination—sometimes with chickenpox added—was the first vaccine to incorporate multiple live virus strains.[42] This combined shot eases the logistics of vaccine delivery, especially in developing countries where follow-up booster shots are often missed.[43] Issues of storage and refrigeration are critical in developing countries;[44] the MMR vaccine can be stored at room temperature or in a refrigerator, so long as it is not exposed to light or allowed to freeze;[45] conversely, the live-virus chickenpox vaccine must be stored frozen, which limits its availability in many parts of the world.[46]

The refined measles vaccine is weaker than the original, providing slightly less protection but with almost no side effects.[47] Whereas measles infection provides lifelong immunity against recurrence of symptoms, vaccination provides less than that—which makes sense, since the body is given less measles.[48] Immunity from vaccination lasts about 20 years, although in regions where measles is still prevalent, that immunity lasts longer in practice, as vaccinated individuals are "boosted" by subsequent infections that they don't notice.[49]

The measles vaccine heralded a cultural shift in attitudes towards vaccines as a public-health tool.[50] Political leadership in support of immunization at the local level grew substantially, while immunization proponents championed mandatory vaccination of children as the best means of ensuring a protected population.[51] This support for vaccination coincided with the age of television, because producers at CBS in 1963 wanted to dramatize the development of two new measles vaccines and detail the disease's toll in West Africa.[52] Their production cemented the idea that mass vaccinations could not only help manage infectious diseases but actually eradicate them, selling the measles vaccine as a triumph of Western medicine.[53] Immunization programs were extended to the "mild" childhood diseases like measles, because they were seen as less severe than previous targets of mass vaccination such as smallpox, polio, or diphtheria.[54]

Before the widespread use of the vaccine, measles was so common that infection was considered as inevitable as death and taxes.[55] Despite its high transmissibility, the vaccination program in North America was so successful that measles was declared eliminated from the continent in the year 2000.[56] Elimination status is achieved when more than 12 months have passed without transmission. However, with elimination comes the loss of immunity, since there is no circulating measles to provide an immune boost.

It should be noted that measles mortality was falling before the introduction of the vaccine, in part due to the reduction in malnourished children.[57] Measles, along with resulting pneumonia and encephalitis complications, increases in severity in children lacking in vitamin A. The importance of vitamin A in preventing death from measles was a chance discovery during a randomized trial of vitamin A to prevent eye disease.[58]

Despite huge success in the richer parts of the world, measles is not gone. Even with a vaccine, fatality rates are as still high as 28% in developing countries with poor healthcare.[59] Measles remains the number one cause of death among vaccine-preventable diseases. And, despite the success in North America at the beginning of the twenty-first century, measles sadly came back to the continent.[60] With such high transmissibility, it's easy for an imported measles case to spark a new outbreak, especially among unvaccinated individuals.[61] Not everyone can get vaccinated; some people have compromised immune systems or severe allergies that make them unable to tolerate vaccines.[62] These people rely on herd immunity: sufficiently many people around them being vaccinated so that the disease can't reach them.[63] However, there's another problem, which has expanded in recent years: anti-vaxxers.

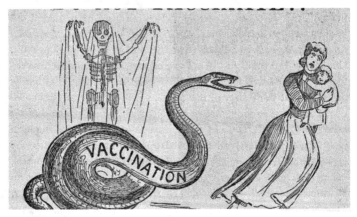

Figure 4.2. A cartoon from a December 1894 anti-vaccination publication.
Source: The Historical Medical Library of the College of Physicians of Philadelphia, December 1894.

Anti-vaxxers are nothing new; they've been around as long as there have been vaccines. Anti-vaxxers essentially work like parasites: a small number can be tolerated, but too many and the system collapses.[64] Childhood vaccinations are particularly susceptible to anti-vax rhetoric, with a number of parents who are not necessarily anti-vaxxers but *vaccine hesitant.*[65] This refers to people who do not vaccinate but are potentially persuadable.[66] We'll discuss the anti-vax movement more in chapter 3.

In many ways, vaccines are a victim of their own success. When epidemics are raging, people tend to vaccinate (not always, as COVID-19 shows, but most do). Once an epidemic is under control, vaccination often continues for a generation, as cultural memory of the disease remains.[67] However, it then loosens, as people are reluctant to vaccinate against a disease they haven't experienced for themselves. This can be okay for a time, but it creates a crucible of susceptible individuals. And with a high R_0, such as measles possesses, it only takes a small spark to restart the fire.

This is exactly what happened in Disneyland in 2014. Vaccination rates among school children in some places in California were extremely low. At Berkeley Rose School in Alameda County, only 13% of kindergarten students were up to date on vaccinations. George De La Torre Jr. Elementary in Los Angeles was similar, at 14%.[68] Schools were required to enforce proof of vaccination, but loopholes based on "personal belief exemptions" (either religious beliefs or fear of vaccine injury) or conditional vaccination (promises to be vaccinated in future) were available.[69] However, an outbreak of measles in the Anaheim theme park quickly spread among children, with 125 symptomatic cases, although fortunately no deaths. This resulted in an overhaul of the Californian school system, which began eliminating the personal-belief exemptions and conditional-vaccination loopholes.[70]

Parents, of course, hated it. There were protests in the streets. However, crucially, they did it. Faced with the alternative of home schooling, parents got their kids vaccinated.[71] Reluctantly and under protest perhaps, but they did it. Vaccination rates jumped to more than 90% within a few years. Concerns that parents would pull their kids out of schools never materialized, while only a very few fake medical exemptions were substituted for belief exemptions.[72]

The lessons for COVID-19 vaccination are clear. Some people don't like vaccinations—the best strategy is for everyone else to be vaccinated except me, because then I can enjoy herd immunity without getting the needle in the first place, which of course entirely fails if everyone thinks the same way—but vaccines are part of the social contract: the price we pay for living in a society. They're a bit like taxes: nobody actually enjoys them, but the alternative is much, much worse. Requiring proof of vaccination for restaurants, movie theatres, et cetera means that the vaccine hesitant will get the shot, even if some diehard anti-vaxxers still won't.[73]

One of the misleading things about vaccines is that every side effect must be reported, whether it's caused by the vaccine or not.[74] So if grandpa was about to die of a heart attack tomorrow anyway but got the vaccine today, his heart attack is listed as a side effect. It doesn't mean the vaccine caused his heart attack, but it is tracked. This is correlation, which is not the same as causation, but the two are often confused, especially by the anti-vax movement.[75]

Vaccines are one of the most amazing things humans have ever invented. Life expectancy has doubled in a century—it was 45 in England in 1900, then the richest nation on Earth; it's now 83—in part thanks to vaccination (clean water, food abundance, and a drop in infant mortality were the other factors).[76] Thanks to people like Maurice Hilleman, a great many of us are alive today because of vaccines. But there's an even bigger achievement for which they're responsible, one we'll see in the next chapter.

Notes

1. M. J. Mina, "Measles, Immune Suppression and Vaccination: Direct and Indirect Nonspecific Vaccine Benefits," *Journal of Infection* 74 (2017): S10–S17.
2. W. Yang, "Transmission Dynamics of and Insights from the 2018–2019 Measles Outbreak in New York City: A Modeling Study," *Science Advances* 6, no. 22 (2020): eaaz4037.
3. J. S. Warrack, "The Differential Diagnosis of Scarlet Fever, Measles, and Rubella," *British Medical Journal* 2, no. 3018 (1918): 486–488.
4. R. D. Semba and M. W. Bloem, "Measles Blindness," *Survey of Ophthalmology* 49, no. 2 (2004): 243–255.
5. A. Düx et al., "Measles Virus and Rinderpest Virus Divergence Dated to the Sixth Century BCE," *Science* 368, no. 6497 (2020): 1367–1370.
6. P. Wohlsein and J. Saliki, "Rinderpest and Peste des Petits Ruminants—The Diseases: Clinical Signs and Pathology," in *Rinderpest and Peste des Petits Ruminants*, ed. T. Barrett, P.-P. Pastoret, and W. Taylor (London: Academic Press, 2006), 68–85.

7. M. Wayne and B. Bolker, *Infectious Diseases: A Very Short Introduction* (Oxford: Oxford University Press, 2015).

8. A. Düx et al., "Measles Virus and Rinderpest Virus Divergence Dated to the Sixth Century BCE."

9. B. A. Jones et al., "Zoonosis Emergence Linked to Agricultural Intensification and Environmental Change," *Proceedings of the National Academy of Sciences* 110 (2013): 8399–8404.

10. B. Dalfardi, G. S. Nezhad, and A. Ghanizadeh, "Rhazes' Description of a Case with Aortic Regurgitation," *International Journal of Cardiology* 172, no. 1 (2014): e147–148.

11. E. F. Torrey and R. H. Yolken, "Their Bugs Are Worse Than Their Bite," *The Washington Post*, 3 April 2005.

12. J. C. Bester, "Measles and Measles Vaccination: A Review," *Journal of the American Medical Association Pediatrics* 170, no. 12 (2016): 1209–1215.

13. S. K. Kabra and R. Lodha, "Antibiotics for Preventing Complications in Children with Measles," *Cochrane Database of Systematic Reviews* 8, article CD001477 (2013).

14. D. E. Griffin, W. H. Lin, and C. H. Pan, "Measles Virus, Immune Control, and Persistence," *FEMS Microbiology Reviews* 36, no. 3 (2012): 649–662.

15. I. K. Kouadio, T. Kamigaki, and H. Oshitani, "Measles Outbreaks in Displaced Populations: A Review of Transmission, Morbidity and Mortality Associated Factors," *BMC International Health and Human Rights* 10 (2010): 5.

16. K. Dietz, "The Estimation of the Basic Reproduction Number for Infectious Diseases," *Statistical Methods in Medical Research* 2, no. 1 (1993): 23–41.

17. P. L. Delamater et al., "Complexity of the Basic Reproduction Number (R_0)," *Emerging Infectious Diseases* 25, no. 1 (2019): 1–4.

18. J. Li, D. Blakeley, and R.J. Smith?, "The Failure of R_0," *Computational and Mathematical Methods in Medicine* article 527610 (2011).

19. R. Breban, R., Vardavas, and S. Blower, "Theory Versus Data: How to Calculate R_0?," *PLoS ONE* 2, no. 3 (2007): e282.

20. C. Costris-Vas, E.J. Schwartz, and R. Smith?, "Predicting COVID-19 Using Past Pandemics as a Guide: How Reliable Were Mathematical Models Then, and How Reliable Will They Be Now?," *Mathematical Biosciences and Engineering* 17, no. 6 (2020): 7502–7518.

21. Y. Liu and J. Rocklöv, "The Reproductive Number of the Delta Variant of SARS-CoV-2 Is Far Higher Compared to the Ancestral SARS-CoV-2 Virus," *Journal of Travel Medicine* 28, no. 7 (2021): 1–3.

22. M. Weisberger, "This One Number Shows Why Measles Spreads like Wildfire," *Live Science*, 8 February 2019.

23. P. P. Rubió, "Is the Basic Reproductive Number (R_0) for Measles Viruses Observed in Recent Outbreaks Lower than in the Pre-Vaccination Era?," *Eurosurveillance* 17, no. 31 (2021): pi=20233.

24. Y. Liu and J. Rocklöv, "The Effective Reproductive Number of the Omicron Variant of SARS-CoV-2 Is Several Times Relative to Delta," *Journal of Travel Medicine* 29, no. 3 (2022): taac037.

25. W. Moss, "Measles in Vaccinated Individuals and the Future of Measles Elimination," *Clinical Infectious Diseases* 67, no. 9 (2018): 1320–1321.

26. S. C. Alumona, "Globalisation and Disease Spread in the World: Review from Socio-Cultural Perspective," *International Journal of Health and Social Inquiry* 1, no. 1 (2011).

27. R. Dagan et al., "Marking November 12, 2010—World Pneumonia Day: Where Are We, Where Are Vaccines?," *Human Vaccines* 6, no. 11 (2010): 922–925.

28. D. C. Morley, "Measles in the Developing World," *Proceedings of the Royal Society of Medicine* 67 (1974): 1112–1115.

29. S. T. Shulman, D. L. Shulman, and R. H. Sims, "The Tragic 1824 journey of the Hawaiian King and Queen to London: History of Measles in Hawaii," *The Pediatric Infectious Disease Journal* 28, no. 8 (2009): 728–733.

30. H. Hall, "The SkepDoc: Mark Twain and Alternative Medicine," *Skeptic* 26, no. 2 (2021): 4–7.

31. J. C. Moore and J. A. Brylinsky, "Spectator Effect on Team Performance in College Basketball," *Journal of Sport Behavior* 16, no. 2 (1993): 77–85.

32. D. W. Davies, "Dahl and Dylan: Matilda,'In Country Sleep' and Twentieth-Century Topographies of Fear," in *Roald Dahl: Wales of the Unexpected*, ed. D.W. Davies (Cardiff: University of Wales Press, 2016), 91–118.

33. J. P. Baker, "The First Measles Vaccine," *Pediatrics* 128, no. 3 (2011): 435–437.

34. S. Krugman, "Further-Attenuated Measles Vaccine: Characteristics and Use," *Reviews of Infectious Diseases* 5, no. 3 (1983): 477–481.

35. M. R. Hilleman, "Past, Present, and Future of Measles, Mumps, and Rubella Virus Vaccines," *Pediatrics* 90, no. 1 (1992): 149–153.

36. L. Newman, "Maurice Hilleman," *British Medical Journal* 330, no. 7498 (2005): 1028.

37. T. J. Tulchinsky, "Maurice Hilleman: Creator of Vaccines that Changed the World," *Case Studies in Public Health* (2018): 443–470.

38. M. K. Slifka and I. J. Amanna, "Vaccinated: One Man's Quest to Defeat the World's Deadliest Diseases," *Journal of the American Medical Association* 298, no. 16 (2007): 1943–1949.

39. N. Escobar, "You Should Thank Maurice Hilleman for Helping You Live Past the Age of 10," *Smithsonian Magazine*, 25 October 2017.

40. A. Harding, "Vaccine Maker," *The Lancet* 370, no. 9593 (2007): 1120.

41. A. Dove, "Maurice Hilleman," *Nature Medicine* 11, no. 4 (2005): S2.

42. M. Knuf et al., "A Combination Vaccine against Measles, Mumps, Rubella and Varicella," *Drugs of Today* 44, no. 4 (2008): 279–292.

43. K. Maman et al., "The Value of Childhood Combination Vaccines: From Beliefs to Evidence," *Human Vaccines & Immunotherapeutics* 11, no. 9 (2015): 2132–2141.

44. M. M. Levine and R. Robins-Browne, "Vaccines, Global Health and Social Equity," *Immunology and Cell Biology* 87, no. 4 (2009): 274–278.

45. S. Ohtake et al., "Heat-Stable Measles Vaccine Produced by Spray Drying," *Vaccine* 28, no. 5 (2010): 1275–1284.

46. G. Laustsen and T. Neilson, "Prevent Shingles with Zostavax," *The Nurse Practitioner* 32, no. 6 (2007): 6–7.

47. M. K. Slifka and I. Amanna, "How Advances in Immunology Provide Insight into Improving Vaccine Efficacy," *Vaccine* 32, no. 25 (2014): 2948–2957.

48. J. Mossong and C. P. Muller, "Modelling Measles Re-Emergence as a Result of Waning of Immunity in Vaccinated Populations," *Vaccine* 21, no. 31 (2003): 4597–4603.

49. D. Güris et al., "Measles Vaccine Effectiveness and Duration of Vaccine-Induced Immunity in the Absence of Boosting from Exposure to Measles Virus," *The Pediatric Infectious Disease Journal* 15, no. 12 (1996): 1082–1086.

50. C. J. Clements and F. T. Cutts, "The Epidemiology of Measles: Thirty Years of Vaccination," in *Measles Virus*, ed. V. Meulen and M. A. Billeter (Berlin: Springer-Verlag, 1995), 13–33.

51. E. Conis, "Measles and the Modern History of Vaccination," *Public Health Reports* 134 (2019): 118–125.

52. J. S. Hunter and B. E. Becker, "Telling the World about Measles: Case History in Government Information," *Public Health Reports* 78 (1963): 893–896.

53. J. P. Baker, "Immunization and the American Way: 4 Childhood Vaccines," *American Journal of Public Health* 90, no. 2 (2000): 199–207.

54. E. Conis, "Measles and the Modern History of Vaccination".

55. F. L. Babbott and J. E. Gordon, "Modern Measles," *The American Journal of the Medical Sciences* 228 (1954): 334–361.

56. W. A. Orenstein, A. R. Hinman, and M. J. Papania, "Evolution of Measles Elimination Strategies in the United States," *The Journal of Infectious Diseases* 189, suppl. 1 (2004): S17–S22.

57. P. Aaby, "Malnutrition and Overcrowding/Intensive Exposure in Severe Measles Infection: Review of Community Studies," *Clinical Infectious Diseases* 10, no. 2 (1988): 478–491.

58. H. M. Yang, M. Mao, and C. Wan, "Vitamin A for Treating Measles in Children," *Cochrane Database of Systematic Reviews* 2005, no. 4 (2005): CD001479.

59. N. A. Halsey, "Increased Mortality after High Titer Measles Vaccines: Too Much of a Good Thing," *The Pediatric Infectious Disease Journal* 12, no. 6 (1993): 462–465.

60. J. C. Bester, "Measles and Measles Vaccination: A Review," *Journal of the American Medical Association Pediatrics* 170 (2016): 1209–1215.

61. J. M. Ochoche and R. I. Gweryina, "A Mathematical Model of Measles with Vaccination and Two Phases of Infectiousness," *IOSR Journal of Mathematics* 10, no. 1 (2014): 95–105.

62. J. C. Bester, "The Ethical Obligation to Vaccinate Children and Its Policy Implications," *Journal for Research and Debate* 3, no. 8 (2020): 1–5.

63. B. Ashby and A. Best, "Herd Immunity," *Current Biology* 31, no. 4 (2021): R174–R177.

64. R. Baker, "The Dangers of Vaccine Hesitancy," *The Write Path* 4 (2020): 25–31.

65. M. Badar, "Calling the Shots: Balancing Parental and Child Rights in the Age of Anti-Vax," *Indiana Journal of Global Legal Studies* 28, no. 1 (2021): 325–348.

66. D. J. Opel et al., "Development of a Survey to Identify Vaccine-Hesitant Parents: The Parent Attitudes about Childhood Vaccines Survey," *Human Vaccines* 7, no. 4 (2011): 419–425.

67. D. S. Saint-Victor and S. B. Omer, "Vaccine Refusal and the Endgame: Walking the Last Mile First," *Philosophical Transactions of the Royal Society B: Biological Sciences* 368, no. 1623 (2013): 20120148.

68. E. Oster and G. Kocks, "After a Debacle, How California Became a Role Model on Measles," *The New York Times*, 16 January 2018.

69. E. Wang et al., "Nonmedical Exemptions from School Immunization Requirements: A Systematic Review," *American Journal of Public Health* 104, no. 11 (2014): e62–e84.

70. D. A. Broniatowski, K. M. Hilyard, and M. Dredze, "Effective Vaccine Communication during the Disneyland Measles Outbreak," *Vaccine* 34, no. 28 (2016): 3225–3228.

71. P. McDonald et al., "Exploring California's New Law Eliminating Personal Belief Exemptions to Childhood Vaccines and Vaccine Decision-Making among Homeschooling Mothers in California," *Vaccine* 37, no. 5 (2019): 742–750.

72. E. Oster and G. Kocks, "After a Debacle, How California Became a Role Model on Measles."

73. L. O. Gostin, D. A. Salmon, and H. J. Larson, "Mandating COVID-19 Vaccines," *Journal of the American Medical Association* 325, no. 6 (2021): 532–533.

74. A. Di Pasquale et al., "Vaccine Safety Evaluation: Practical Aspects in Assessing Benefits and Risks," *Vaccine* 34, no. 52 (2016): 6672–6680.

75. D. Jolley and K. M. Douglas, "The Effects of Anti-Vaccine Conspiracy Theories on Vaccination Intentions," *PloS ONE* 9, no. 2 (2014): e89177.

76. M. Roser, E. Ortiz-Ospina, and H. Ritchie, "Life Expectancy," *Our World in Data*, 2013, https://ourworldindata.org/life-expectancy (accessed 4 June 2022).

3 Smallpox

For many millennia, having children was the only way to ensure your future. They helped manage farms and supported you in your old age (assuming you made it that far). That was one of the reasons people had so many children back in the day, but another was because smallpox was likely to kill a fair number of them.

Like Ebola, SARS, and COVID-19, smallpox is thought to have originated in bats.[1] However, it's difficult to be sure, because it likely emerged somewhere around 16,000–68,000 years ago, when we became agriculturalists, as estimated by phylogenetic genome analysis.[2] The first recorded instance of smallpox is in the New Kingdom of Egypt, which lasted from 1550–1069 BCE.[3] Ancient Sanskrit medical texts dated 1500 BCE describe an infection with pustules that were identical to the form of smallpox seen in the twentieth century,[4] and one of the pharaohs, Ramesses V, died from it in 1157 BCE.[5]

Symptoms of smallpox included fever, vomiting, mouth ulcers, and a telltale skin rash. Survivors had extensive scarring, and some were left blind.[6] It was an airborne disease, being transmitted similarly to COVID-19, with prolonged face-to-face contact between two people within six feet or by contact with fomites* or bodily fluids.[7] An individual with smallpox remained infectious until the last scab had healed.[8]

There were two forms most commonly seen: variola major and variola minor.[9] The former was the most common type and by far the most lethal, with a case-fatality rate of around 30%. The latter was milder and fatal in less than 1% of cases.[10] Two rare forms also existed: hemorrhagic and malignant, both of which were invariably fatal.[11]

However, surviving smallpox was no picnic either. It caused blindness, disfigurement, and sterility, although at least it had the advantage of conferring permanent immunity.[12] Because of this immunity, survivors were often called upon to nurse victims back to health. "Treatment" often involved bloodletting, herbal remedies, and exposing people to red objects.[13]

However, the reason we're talking about smallpox in the past tense is because—famously—it's gone. (Well, almost.) The disease was declared

---

* Fomites are objects or materials—such as clothes, utensils, and furniture—that carry infection.

eradicated in 1980 by the World Health Organization, in what stands as one of the pinnacles of human achievement.[14] It is the only human disease ever to be eradicated[15] and one of only two that we've managed to fight to zero (the other being rinderpest, the cattle plague discussed in chapters 4 and 5).[16] The road to eradication was long and fraught, and it has lessons for us as we fight other diseases, including COVID-19.

Before we wiped it out, smallpox killed *300–500 million* people—and that was in the twentieth century alone.[17] Before that, smallpox was responsible for a whopping 8%–20% of all deaths in Europe.[18] Smallpox had the twin advantages of being very transmissible and very lethal, whereas most diseases tend to lean either in one direction or another. If a disease is too lethal, it kills the host before it can be passed on. Smallpox was in the sweet spot of a high case-fatality rate and high transmissibility.[19]

One of the reasons it was so successful at transmitting itself around the world was because of innovations in global trade and movement.[20] In the sixth century, increased trade with China and Korea brought the disease to Japan.[21] Seventh-century Arab expansion brought it to Northern Africa, Spain, and Portugal.[22] The Crusades spread smallpox throughout Europe in the eleventh century. European settlers and the African slave trade brought smallpox to the Caribbean and to Central and South America in the sixteenth century, while European settlers brought it to North America in the seventeenth century, and the British took it to Australia in the eighteenth.[23]

Smallpox was particularly effective whenever it encountered virgin soil: places where no disease had gone before, with populations correspondingly having no immunity. When smallpox hit Iceland in 1707, it killed nearly a third of the population in two years. A similar epidemic ravaged the Khoisan people of South Africa in 1713.[24]

History is littered with the victims of smallpox. In the seventeenth and eighteenth centuries, it killed several reigning European monarchs, including Habsburg Emperor Joseph I; Queen Mary II of England, Scotland, and Ireland; Czar Peter II of Russia; King Louis XV of France; Negasi Krestos, a ruling prince of Ethiopia; King Boranarja IV of Siam; and the Japanese emperor Go-Kōmyō.[25] There are also many famous names among the survivors. Abraham Lincoln contracted it shortly before giving the Gettysburg Address. The severity was downplayed by his doctor to prevent the public from worrying the president was dying, but he was dizzy and haggard during the speech and likely infected his valet afterwards, who died from the disease.[26] Andrew Jackson, future U.S. president, contracted smallpox at age 14 while being held prisoner by the British during the Revolutionary War. Queen Elizabeth I survived it,[27] but it left her scarred, resulting in her wearing the white face makeup seen in all portraits; the lead base in its foundation is thought to have eventually killed her.[28]

Smallpox was also responsible for the Plague of Athens in 430 BCE, which killed 100,000 people, and the Antonine Plague of 165–180 CE, which killed 3.5–7 million people, including Emperor Marcus Aurelius.[29] Upon reaching the Americas, it tore through the native populations, killing up to 90%, including many of the Aztecs, along with their second-to-last ruler.[30] The disease first appeared in Brazil in 1563 and caused the extermination of whole tribes.[31] In North America, the Anishinaabe-speaking Monsoni, powerful middlemen in the beaver trade of the 1670s, were decimated by smallpox in the 1730s; survivors drifted to other groups and ceased to be a discrete people by the end of the century.[32] It was so prevalent and fearsome that some cultures worshipped smallpox deities.[33]

Not all these infections occurred by chance. Lord Jeffrey Amherst, the commander-in-chief of British forces in North America during the French and Indian War, advocated handing out smallpox-infected blankets to his Native American foes in 1763.[34] There is no evidence that this was acted upon, but there is a single documented case that precedes this: the British gave gifts of two blankets and a handkerchief that had come from the small-pox ward,[35] with their commander writing "I hope that it will have the desired effect."

What that desire actually was is open to debate. The smallpox blankets were old, and the virus did not last long on surfaces, so no epidemic resulted from this action.[36] Some have interpreted this statement as a desire to commit genocide, à la Amherst. Others have argued that the desire here was to foster peace through gifts. After all, smallpox had already swept through the native population (and the soldiers) by this time, so anyone who had survived it would have already been immune.[37]

Innumerable people lived in terror of smallpox across the world and searched for some kind of mitigation or prevention. For centuries, there was a technique that worked—sometimes. Variolation involved scraping a smallpox scar and a susceptible person inhaling the particles.[38] This would of course give them smallpox, but in a milder form, so death rates were not as high. It was first practised in China in the fifteenth century,[39] then spread to the Ottoman Empire in 1670.[40] In 1768, Catherine the Great was the first person to receive it in Russia, declaring inoculation skeptics "truly blockheads, ignorant or just wicked."[41] Her embracing of the procedure led to a mass campaign,[42] with over two million Russians inoculated by the end of the century.[43]

Cotton Mather, a Puritan minister who supported the Salem witch trials, was the first proponent of variolation in the United States.[44] Benjamin Franklin lost his child to smallpox and later became an advo-cate of variolation.[45] However, although the death rate was lower than regular smallpox, it was still quite high—about a tenth as high as the mor-tality from the naturally acquired disease—causing many people to refuse it. A variolated person could also transmit virulent smallpox to others.[46] Mandatory inoculation against smallpox was the most significant medi-cal success of the Revolutionary War, and it contributed substantially to America's victory.[47]

The breakthrough came in 1796, when British physician Edward Jenner made an enormous discovery: he noticed that milkmaids were strikingly beautiful.[48] In particular, they had clear skin, unravaged by the scars of smallpox.[49] A milkmaid told him that she would be protected from smallpox because she'd caught cowpox, a related virus in cows that was relatively mild and non-fatal in humans.[50]

Jenner had the idea to deliberately infect people with cowpox and see if it protected them from smallpox.[51] He tried this out on a small boy, his gardener's son, infecting the ten-year-old lad with cowpox and then, some months later, exposing the child to smallpox. (Medical ethics were a bit lax back then.) The child survived, with no symptoms. Jenner experimented on further children, including his 11-month-old son.[52] Due to its cowpox origin, this process was named *vaccine*, after the Latin word for cow (*vacca*).[53]

Jenner's idea would revolutionise medicine and (eventually) put paid to one of the worst scourges our species has ever seen. However, it didn't happen overnight, and it wasn't widely embraced at first.

With the first vaccine came anti-vaxxers. One of the first group of anti-vaxxers were doctors, who felt that treating the sick was their livelihood, so Jenner's vaccine was going to put them out of business.[54] The Royal Society told Jenner not to propagate such wild ideas if he valued his reputation. Fortunately, he ignored them, devoting the rest of his life to vaccinating people against smallpox, including in his own backyard.[55] Eventually, doctors were brought on board for the idea of vaccines, but this took a generation to achieve.[56]

Throughout the nineteenth century, vaccination slowly grew in popularity, but there was of course pushback. The cycle of acceptance tended to have four phases: 1) people dying of smallpox; 2) people embracing the vaccine as a lifeline; 3) cases going down, people keep vaccinating; 4) with no cases for many years, people stop vaccinating.[57] After many years of steady oscillations, major outbreaks in 1838 and 1871 were followed by epidemics with decaying amplitude.[58]

Because of the vaccine's bovine origins, people in the nineteenth century were afraid of giving birth to half human/half cow hybrids. (There were even political cartoons in newspapers depicting this.)[59] Vaccine-induced therianthropes sound as ridiculous to us as the myths of vaccines causing autism or of 5G technology giving you COVID-19 no doubt will to our descendants.

Vaccination wasn't always received negatively. Those who imported the smallpox vaccine to Japan were in the vanguard of opening the country to the West.[60] Vaccination became a principal conduit to modernity, with Japanese physicians using traditional strategies involving scholarship, marriage, and adoption to forge local, national, and international networks to transmit Jenner's vaccine throughout the country.[61]

The twentieth century saw smallpox numbers decline as vaccination slowly spread.[62] A freeze-dried vaccine was developed in the 1940s, meaning that deploying the vaccine to tropical climates became feasible.[63] Countries started to be declared smallpox-free, then whole continents.[64] However, as the disease receded, so did the political will for vaccination. The United States stopped routine vaccination of children in 1971 because an important threshold had been crossed: more children—six to eight per year—were now dying from vaccine complications than from smallpox.[65] Global travel—and especially with the rise of far quicker air travel—then brought infected people in contact with societies that had never experienced smallpox or where smallpox had previously been eliminated.

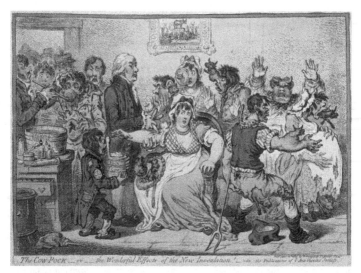

Figure 3.1. British satirist James Gillray caricatured a scene at the Smallpox and Inoculation Hospital at St. Pancras, showing the cowpox vaccine being administered to frightened young women, and cows emerging from different parts of people's bodies. Published by one of the publications of the Anti-Vaccine Society.

Source: H. Humphrey St. James's Street, 12 June 1802.

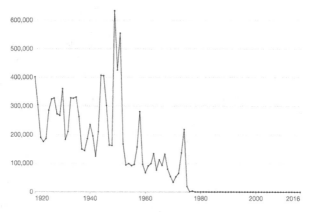

Figure 3.2. Global smallpox numbers 1920–2016.
Source: Our World in Data.

On Christmas Day 1961, five travellers from Pakistan arrived in the United Kingdom, unknowingly infected with smallpox. One travelled to Cardiff, causing an outbreak in Wales. A contact of another travelled to Bradford, resulting in a second outbreak, with every hospital in the city dealing with infected patients.[66] Nineteen people died, and 900,000 people had to be vaccinated in Wales[67] with another 250,000 needing the vaccination as a result of the outbreak in Bradford.[68] The media attention was considerable, with headlines such as "City in Fear!" screaming across the newspapers,[69] and racial tensions were high, due to the country of origin of the travellers.[70]

By the 1970s, smallpox was all but gone.[71] It was considered eradicated in Europe, but a Yugoslavian cleric returning from the Hajj brought it back from Iraq, triggering an outbreak in 1972.[72] Although the population of the former Yugoslavia had been regularly vaccinated for the preceding 50 years (and the last case reported in 1930), an outbreak erupted across Kosovo province, leading to 175 infections and 35 deaths.[73] Government reaction was to declare martial law, isolating whole villages and using hotels to quarantine 10,000 people under armed guard.[74] A mass re-vaccination of the population was undertaken, with almost the entire country vaccinated—an astonishing 18 million people in a little over a month.[75]

The last person to acquire natural occurring variola major was Rahima Banu, a three-year-old girl from a Bangladeshi island, in late 1975.[76] She was isolated at home and guards posted 24 hours a day until she was no longer infected.[77] A vaccination campaign of every house within a 1.5-mile radius was undertaken, and members of the WHO Smallpox Eradication Program visited every house, school, and healer on the island to ensure the disease did not spread, offering a reward to anyone who reported a case of smallpox.[78] Rahima survived (and is still alive) but she wasn't quite the last person to catch the disease.

The last person to acquire variola minor was Ali Maow Maalin, a hospital cook in Somalia who rode in a vehicle with two smallpox patients from the hospital to the local smallpox office on October 12, 1977.[79] The journey took about ten minutes, and the six-year-old girl who died, Habiba Nur Ali, was the last person to die from naturally acquired smallpox. Maalin was diagnosed with smallpox and then isolated but made a full recovery. He went on to work on the measles-vaccination and polio-eradication campaigns and eventually died of malaria in 2013.[80] Maalin was the last person infected with naturally occurring smallpox, but there was one more outbreak.

In 1978, Janet Parker, a medical photographer at Birmingham University's medical school, contracted smallpox after working one floor above the Medical Microbiology Department, where staff and students were conducting smallpox research.[81] She became ill on August 11 and died on September 11, 1978, the last person to die from a disease that had killed so many millions. Her mother, who was caring for her, developed smallpox on September 7, despite having received the vaccine two weeks earlier, although she survived.[82] (Her father did not, dying of a cardiac arrest after visiting his daughter, whereas the head of the Medical Microbiology Department committed suicide while in quarantine.)[83] The subsequent inquiry triggered radical changes in how dangerous pathogens would be stored and studied.[84]

In the late 1970s, the World Health Organization scoured the planet for any traces of the disease but found none.[85] Smallpox thus took the honour of the first—and so far last—human disease to be eradicated. There's some debate about whether we eradicated SARS, as no cases have been seen since 2004, but it's difficult to definitively say whether a zoonotic disease can ever truly be said to be eradicated.[86]

Table 3.1. Year of smallpox eradication in selected countries

Country	Year of final natural occurring smallpox case
Iceland	1872
Sweden	1895
Norway	1898
French Guiana	1904
New Zealand	1914
Australia	1917
United States	1948
Portugal	1953
Yugoslavia	1972
Bangladesh	1975
Ethiopia	1976
Kenya	1977
Somalia	1977

Source: A. O'Neill, "Number of Countries where Smallpox Was Eradicated in Nature 1872–1977," *Statista* (12 June 2022).

Back in 1002 CE, in response to Viking attacks, King Æthelred the Unready ordered all Danes in England to be executed. They were rounded up at what is now St John's College Oxford and murdered in the St Brice Day massacre. Some of them had smallpox. Fast forward to 2020 and DNA evidence from these skeletons revealed that there was a different, long-extinct, strain of smallpox present among the victims.[87] This version was less lethal and had a common ancestor with the strain that Jenner eradicated, which overturned the common assumption that viruses get less deadly over time.[88] This also means that smallpox has the distinction of being not just the only disease to go extinct, but also the only one to do so twice.

Four diseases were targeted for eradication in the twentieth century: smallpox, malaria, yellow fever, and yaws.[89] These diseases were chosen based on medical advances, such as newly available treatments, vaccines, or insecticides. We'll discuss malaria shortly. Despite an excellent vaccine, yellow fever could not be eradicated due to animal reservoirs, which had not been known to exist.[90] Eliminating a disease in humans is challenging enough, but it's almost impossible to do so in animal populations (at least without exterminating all the animals), and the disease can simply start over by jumping across species again.[91] Yaws, a tropical infection of the skin and bone, was significantly reduced, but the strategy changed from one of active eradication to a surveillance campaign when numbers fell, which failed to maintain the required pressure; it was also found that asymptomatic cases were far more prevalent than previously believed.[92] This lapse in aggressive pursuit of the disease meant that eradication was not achieved, although efforts are still ongoing, with India declared yaws-free in 2016.[93]

There are two more diseases whose eradication may be on the horizon: polio and Guinea-worm disease.[94] The push for polio eradication was very strong, since the disease has been eliminated from all countries except Afghanistan and Pakistan.[95] (Queen Elizabeth II vaccinating her children against polio in the 1950s was instrumental in raising acceptance of childhood vaccinations in much of the world.)[96] However, resistance to polio vaccination as a U.S. tool of imperialism grew in Pakistan following Osama bin Laden's execution: Navy SEAL troops infiltrated his compound after a pretext of polio vaccination was used to positively identify bin Laden's family in 2011.[97] Consequently, polio numbers doubled in 2014, and hopes for full eradication have dwindled.[98]

The polio-eradication program was so successful that the disease is mostly gone in the wild, meaning that some of the polio still circulating derives directly from the vaccine—which doesn't help vaccination efforts. Oral polio vaccines cause less than one case of vaccine-associated polio per million doses given,[99] which is tiny compared to the 5,000 cases per million who are paralyzed following infection,[100] but it's not zero. Currently, 15% of circulating polio cases are caused by the vaccine itself, a further roadblock to vaccination.[101] In 2022, vaccine-derived polio was discovered in stool specimens of unvaccinated adults and wastewater in several New York counties.[102]

As mentioned in the introduction, Guinea-worm disease is a non-lethal parasitic infection that used to be widespread. It's mentioned in the Bible, and Egyptian mummies showed signs of it.[103] It's spread through the drinking water (and in fact is the only disease spread solely through drinking water), making the chain of transmission relatively easy to stop.[104] Distribution of cloth filters to villages has been useful, while nomadic people now wear pipes around their necks on strings so that when they come to an unfamiliar water source, they can drink through filters.[105] This helps reduce Guinea-worm transmission, and it's also good for overall health. Chlorination of the water can kill the parasite's host, the water flea.[106] However, the most useful intervention method for Guinea-worm disease is education, because teaching people about the disease's life cycle allows them to change behaviour and break the cycle.[107] With no medical interventions, this achievement speaks to the power of "soft skills"—local education, neighbours talking to neighbours, public–private partnerships—in achieving significant outcomes.[108]

Indeed, during the global smallpox-eradication campaign, the "soft" skills were just as important as the vaccine. Many people did not get vaccinated because they didn't actually know what smallpox was, as it had different local names.[109] A key tool was photographic-recognition cards, showing pictures of someone infected with smallpox in order to determine whether there was smallpox in this village.[110] These efforts require understanding and investing in people, not just technology, which is something the Western world is not typically good at.

We said at the beginning that smallpox was almost gone. What still remains? As the disease was being eradicated, it was argued that some samples should be kept for research purposes.[111] Of course, these arguments were cover for the military, who wanted it as a potential bioweapon (or to defend against one).[112] Initially, four countries kept samples: the United States, the former U.S.S.R., the United Kingdom, and South Africa. Eventually, the United Kingdom and South Africa either destroyed their samples or moved them to one of the other facilities. Currently, smallpox only exists in two known locations: in secure labs in Moscow and Atlanta.[113]

This brings up the question of whether it's ethical to eradicate a disease. It sounds like there's an obvious answer, but the issue is a little more nuanced than it might appear. There are two issues at play. The first is whether we should commit what would technically be genocide against a species or quasi-species. Viruses aren't technically alive, whereas bacteria and parasites are usually not considered to be as worthy of life as other creatures that might threaten us, such as lions or sharks (or even mosquitoes),[114] so few people lose much sleep over their removal. However, sometimes eradicating a pathogen means eradicating its vector—to control sleeping sickness, you have to wipe out the tsetse flies that carry it—and that opens up issues of biodiversity conservation.[115]

The second issue is to do with the impact of a disease on society. At first glance, eradicating a disease would appear to be an obvious goal we can all get behind, but there are complications that get in the way. There are three criteria for the eradication of a disease: 1) biological and technical feasibility; 2) costs and benefits; 3) societal and political considerations.[116] Sometimes it's just not practical to eradicate a disease (for example, if it has animal reservoirs). Sometimes it's just too expensive. And sometimes there are cultural traditions, religious beliefs, and so forth that make disease control difficult in practice (such as funeral practices and Ebola, as mentioned in chapter 9, or conspiracy theories and COVID-19).

After the 9/11 attacks in the United States, there was an outbreak of mail-borne anthrax, prompting fears of other bioweapons, including smallpox.[117] As a result, the United States stockpiled enough smallpox vaccines to inoculate every citizen[118] (something they would not have needed to do if all samples had been destroyed). When the Soviet Union fell, there were fears that the smallpox samples were not safe and might fall into terrorist hands.[119] There was precedent for this fear: the Japanese used plague as a weapon during the Second World War,[120] while the Soviet Union had stockpiled enormous amounts of *Y. pestis* (the bacterium responsible for the plague) in preparation for all-out war.[121]

The 2022 monkeypox outbreak brought smallpox back into the limelight. Monkeypox is closely related to smallpox, so much so that the smallpox vaccine works to prevent monkeypox.[122] Monkeypox was initially identified in 1958 but was unknown outside sub-Saharan Africa until 2003, when a small outbreak in the United States was contained after 71 cases.[123] In 2022, a similar outbreak failed to be contained, spreading worldwide.[124] However, individuals who had been vaccinated against smallpox decades earlier were not found to be immune to monkeypox.[125]

Regardless, the eradication of smallpox from the planet stands as one of humanity's greatest achievements. As early as 1806, U.S. President Thomas Jefferson wrote to Edward Jenner, saying: "You have erased from the calendar of human afflictions one of its greatest. Yours is the comfortable reflection that mankind can never forget that you have lived. Future nations will know by history only that the loathsome small-pox has existed and by you has been extirpated."[126] Happily for all us today, those turned out to be prophetic words.

Notes

1. Z. Wu et al., "Deciphering the Bat Virome Catalog to Better Understand the Ecological Diversity of Bat Viruses and the Bat Origin of Emerging Infectious Diseases," *The ISME Journal* 10, no. 3 (2016): 609–620.

2. Y. Li et al., "On the Origin of Smallpox: Correlating Variola Phylogenics with Historical Smallpox Records," *Proceedings of the National Academy of Sciences USA* 104 (2007): 15787–15792.

3. E. Strouhal, "Traces of a Smallpox Epidemic in the Family of Ramesses V of the Egyptian 20th Dynasty," *Anthropologie* 34, no. 3 (1996): 315–319.

4. A. Khalakdina, A. Costa, and S. Brianda, "Smallpox in the Posteradication Era," *Weekly Epidemiological Record* 91, no. 20 (2016): 257–264.

5. E. Strouhal, "Traces of a Smallpox Epidemic in the Family of Ramesses V of the Egyptian 20th Dynasty".

6. J. M. Lofquist, N. A. Weimert, and M. S. Hayney, "Smallpox: A Review of Clinical Disease and Vaccination," *American Journal of Health-System Pharmacy* 60, no. 8 (2003): 749–756.

7. D. M. Milton, "What Was the Primary Mode of Smallpox Transmission? Implications for Biodefense," *Frontiers in Cellular and Infection Microbiology* 2 (2012): 150.

8. S. D. Nafziger, "Smallpox," *Critical Care Clinics* 21, no. 4 (2005): 739–746.

9. K. R. Dumbell, H. S. Bedson, and E. Rossier, "Laboratory Differentiation between Variola Major and Variola Minor," *Bulletin of the World Health Organization* 25, no. 1 (1961): 73.

10. P. D. Ellner, "Smallpox: Gone but Not Forgotten," *Infection* 26, no. 5 (1998): 263–269.

11. C. M. Constantin et al., "Smallpox: An Update for Nurses," *Biological Research for Nursing* 4, no. 4 (2003): 282–294.

12. P. Ager, C. Worm Hansen, and P. Sandholt Jensen, "Fertility and Early-Life Mortality: Evidence from Smallpox Vaccination in Sweden," *Journal of the European Economic Association* 16, no. 2 (2018): 487–521.

13. R. H. Jackson, *Demographic Change and Ethnic Survival among the Sedentary Populations on the Jesuit Mission Frontiers of Spanish South America, 1609–1803* (Leiden: Brill, 2015).

14. F. Fenner et al., *Smallpox and Its Eradication* (Geneva: World Health Organization, 1988).

15. W. A. Orenstein and R. Ahmed, "Simply Put: Vaccination Saves Lives," *Proceedings of the National Academy of Sciences* 114, no. 16 (2017): 4031–4033.

16. K. Le Roux, J. Kotze, and K. Perrett, "Elimination of Dog-Mediated Human Rabies: The Burden of Human Rabies in Africa," *Revue Scientifique et Technique* 37, no. 2 (2018): 607–615.

17. P. Berche, "Life and Death of Smallpox," *La Presse Médicale* 51, no. 3 (2022): 104117.

18. F. E. André, "Vaccinology: Past Achievements, Present Roadblocks and Future Promises," *Vaccine* 21, no. 7–8 (2003): 593–595.

19. J. P. Zanders, "Addressing the Concerns about Smallpox," *International Journal of Infectious Diseases* 8 (2004): 9–14.

20. F. Fenner, "Smallpox: Emergence, Global Spread, and Eradication," *History and Philosophy of the Life Sciences* 1 (1993): 397–420.

21. J. Zhang, "Disease and Its Impact on Politics, Diplomacy, and the Military: The Case of Smallpox and the Manchus (1613–1795)," *Journal of the History of Medicine and Allied Sciences* 57, no. 2 (2002): 177–197.

22. S. Riedel, "Edward Jenner and the History of Smallpox and Vaccination," *Baylor University Medical Center Proceedings* 18, no. 1 (2005): 21–25.

23. F. Fenner et al., *Smallpox and Its Eradication*.

24. C. W. McMillen, *Pandemics: A Very Short Introduction* (Oxford: Oxford University Press, 2016).

25. D. R. Hopkins, *The Greatest Killer: Smallpox in History* (Chicago: University of Chicago Press, 2002).

26. A. S. Goldman and F. C. Schmalstieg, "Abraham Lincoln's Gettysburg Illness," *Journal of Medical Biography* 15, no. 2 (2007): 104–110.

27. L. M. Deppisch, "Andrew Jackson and American Medical Practice: Old Hickory and his Physicians," *Tennessee Historical Quarterly* 62, no. 2 (2003): 130–151.

28. L.-J. Charleston, "The Truth behind Queen Elizabeth's White 'Clown Face' Makeup," *Medium*, 12 September 2019.

29. R. J. Littman, "The Plague of Athens: Epidemiology and Paleopathology," *Mount Sinai Journal of Medicine* 76, no. 5 (2009): 456–467.

30. K. Roy and S. Ray, "War and Epidemics: A Chronicle of Infectious Diseases," *Journal of Marine Medical Society* 20, no. 1 (2018): 50–54.

31. A. M. Behbehani, "The Smallpox Story: Life and Death of an Old Disease," *Microbiological Reviews* 47, no. 4 (1983): 455–509.

32. C. W. McMillen, *Pandemics*.

33. R. W. Nicholas, "The Goddess Śītalā and Epidemic Smallpox in Bengal," *The Journal of Asian Studies* 41, no. 1 (November 1981): 21–44.

34. L. S. Mayo, "The Journal of Jeffery Amherst," *The New England Quarterly* 5, no. 3 (1932): 647–650.

35. E. A. Fenn, "Biological Warfare in Eighteenth-Century North America: Beyond Jeffery Amherst," *The Journal of American History* 86, no. 4 (2000): 1552–1580.

36. P. Ranlet, "The British, the Indians, and Smallpox: What Actually Happened at Fort Pitt in 1763?," *Pennsylvania History* 67, no. 3 (2000): 427–441.

37. E. A. Fenn, "Biological Warfare in Eighteenth-Century North America: Beyond Jeffery Amherst".

38. S. Riedel, "Edward Jenner and the History of Smallpox and Vaccination".

39. A. K. C. Leung, "'Variolation' and Vaccination in Late Imperial China, Ca 1570–1911," in *History of Vaccine Development*, ed. S. Plotkin (New York: Springer, 2011), 5–12.

40. S. Riedel, "Edward Jenner and the History of Smallpox and Vaccination".

41. C. Foussianes, "Catherine the Great, Vaccine Queen," *Town & Country*, 2 January 2021.

42. C. P. Schneider and M. D. McDonald, "'The King of Terrors' Revisited: The Smallpox Vaccination Campaign and Its Lessons for Future Biopreparedness," *Journal of Law, Medicine & Ethics* 31, no. 4 (2003): 580–589.

43. C. Foussianes, "Catherine the Great, Vaccine Queen".

44. S. Riedel, "Edward Jenner and the History of Smallpox and Vaccination".

45. M. Best, A. Katamba, and D. Neuhauser, "Making the Right Decision: Benjamin Franklin's Son Dies of Smallpox in 1736," *British Medical Journal Quality & Safety* 16, no. 6 (2007): 478–480.

46. D. A. Henderson, "The Eradication of Smallpox," *Scientific American* 235, no. 4 (1976): 25–33.

47. V. J. Cirillo, "Two Faces of Death: Fatalities from Disease and Combat in America's Principal Wars, 1775 to Present," *Perspectives in Biology and Medicine* 51, no. 1 (2008): 121–133.

48. S. Riedel, "Edward Jenner and the History of Smallpox and Vaccination".

49. B. J. Marshall, "COVID-19 Has Triggered a New Century of Vaccination and Infection Control for the Benefit of All Mankind," *Precision Clinical Medicine* 4, no. 2 (2021): 77–79.

50. N. Barquet and P. Domingo, "Smallpox: The Triumph over the Most Terrible of the Ministers of Death," *Annals of Internal Medicine* 127, no. 8 (1997): 635–642.

51. A. J. Stewart and P. M. Devlin, "The History of the Smallpox Vaccine," *Journal of Infection* 52, no. 5 (2006): 329–334.

52. R. Schils, *How James Watt Invented the Copier: Forgotten Inventions of Our Great Scientists* (New York: Springer, 2012).

53. S. Riedel, "Edward Jenner and the History of Smallpox and Vaccination".

54. I. Amelung, "'Mongols Who Are Not Vaccinated Are Not Permitted to Enter the Capital': Successful Smallpox Prevention and Inoculation in China in the 17th and 18th Centuries," *Forschung Frankfurt* 1.2021 (2021): 23–27.

55. M. A. Faria, "Vaccines (Part I): Jenner, Pasteur, and the Dawn of Scientific Medicine," *Medical Sentinel* 5, no. 2 (2000): 44–48.

56. T. Lanzarotta and M. A. Ramos, "Mistrust in Medicine: The Rise and Fall of America's First Vaccine Institute," *American Journal of Public Health* 108, no. 6 (2018): 741–747.

57. D. S. Saint-Victor and S. B. Omer, "Vaccine Refusal and the Endgame: Walking the Last Mile First," *Philosophical Transactions of the Royal Society B: Biological Sciences* 368, no. 1623 (2013): 20120148.

58. C. J. Duncan, S. R. Duncan, and S. Scott, "Oscillatory Dynamics of Smallpox and the Impact of Vaccination," *Journal of Theoretical Biology* 183, no. 4 (1996): 447–454.

59. C. Nugent, "Hesitancy," *The Southwest Respiratory and Critical Care Chronicles* 9, no. 40 (2021): 69–73.

60. C. W. McMillen, *Pandemics.*

61. A. Jannetta, *The Vaccinators: Smallpox, Medical Knowledge, and the "Opening" of Japan* (Redwood City: Stanford University Press, 2007).

62. J. Banthia and T. Dyson, "Smallpox in Nineteenth-Century India," *Population and Development Review* 25, no. 4 (1999): 649–680.

63. C. W. McMillen, *Pandemics.*

64. S. Barrett, "The Smallpox Eradication Game," *Public Choice* 130, no. 1 (2007): 179–207.

65. C. W. McMillen, *Pandemics.*

66. D. Tovey, "The Bradford Smallpox Outbreak in 1962: A Personal Account," *Journal of the Royal Society of Medicine* 97, no. 5 (2004): 244–247.

67. "1962 South Wales Smallpox Outbreak Memories Recorded," *BBC News*, 12 June 2012.

68. M. I. Meltzer et al., "Modeling Potential Responses to Smallpox as a Bioterrorist Weapon," *Emerging Infectious Diseases* 7, no. 6 (2001): 959–969.

69. D. Tovey, "The Bradford Smallpox Outbreak in 1962: A Personal Account," *Journal of the Royal Society of Medicine* 97, no. 5 (2004): 244–247.

70. R. Bivens, "'The People Have No More Love Left for the Commonwealth': Media, Migration and Identity during the 1961–62 British Smallpox Outbreak," *Immigrants & Minorities* 25, no. 3 (2007): 263–289.

71. A. M. Geddes, "The History of Smallpox," *Clinics in Dermatology* 24, no. 3 (2006): 152–157.

72. B. P. Billauer, "Weapons of Mass Hysteria, Faulty Biothreat Predictions, and Their Impact on National (In) Security: A Case-Study of Smallpox or the Misuse of Mathematical Modeling to Project Biothreats, Terrorism Attacks, and Epidemics," *Health Matrix* 27 (2017): 347–415.

73. L. I. Oztig and O. E. Askin, "Human Mobility and Coronavirus Disease 2019 (COVID-19): A Negative Binomial Regression Analysis," *Public Health* 185 (2020): 364–367.

74. T. V. Inglesby, T. O'Toole, and D. A. Henderson, "Preventing the Use of Biological Weapons: Improving Response Should Prevention Fail," *Clinical Infectious Diseases* 30, no. 6 (2000): 926–929.

75. E. Ristanović et al., "Smallpox as an Actual Biothreat: Lessons Learned from Its Outbreak in x-Yugoslavia in 1972," *Annali Dell Istituto Superiore di Sanita* 52, no. 4 (2016): 587–597.

76. S. O. Foster et al., "Smallpox Eradication in Bangladesh, 1972–1976," *Vaccine* 29 (2011): D22–D29.

77. K. R. Reddy, "Is Smallpox Dead? (The Story of Highly Contagious and Most Feared Disease)," *Journal of Gandaki Medical College-Nepal* 11 (2018): 1.

78. A. M. Geddes, "The History of Smallpox," *Clinics in Dermatology* 24, no. 3 (2006): 152–157.

79. E. A. Ismail, "From Surviving Smallpox to Preventing Measles," *World Health*, 26 July 1988.

80. S. L. Katz, "Polio—New Challenges in 2006," *Journal of Clinical Virology* 36, no. 3 (2006): 163–165.

81. T. O. McGarity, "Contending Approaches to Regulating Laboratory Safety," *Kansas Law Review* 28 (1979): 183–242.

82. M. W. Taylor, *Viruses and Man: A History of Interactions* (Cham: Springer, 2014).

83. B. L. Ligon, "Smallpox: Its History and Reemergence as a Weapon of Biological Warfare," *Seminars in Pediatric Infectious Diseases* 12, no. 1 (2001): 71–80.

84. N. Hawkes, "Small Death in Britain Challenges Presumption of Laboratory Safety: Peer Review Failed Dismally," *Science* 203, no. 4383 (1979): 855–856.

85. E. Hammarlund et al., "Duration of Antiviral Immunity after Smallpox Vaccination," *Nature Medicine* 9, no. 9 (2003): 1131–1137.

86. R. Smith?, "Did We Eradicate SARS? Lessons Learned and the Way Forward," *American Journal of Biomedical Science & Research* 6, no. 2 (2019): 001017.

87. Z. Gorvett, "The Deadly Viruses that Vanished without Trace," *BBC Future*, 21 September 2020.

88. M. Le Page, "DNA from Viking People Reveals the Unexpected History of Smallpox," *New Scientist*, 23 July 2020

89. B. Aylward et al., "When Is a Disease Eradicable? 100 Years of Lessons Learned," *American Journal of Public Health* 90, no. 10 (2000): 1515–1520.

90. F. L. Soper, "Rehabilitation of the Eradication Concept in Prevention of Communicable Diseases," *Public Health Reports* 80, no. 10 (1965): 855–869.

91. S. Sundar and J. Chakravarty, "Leishmaniasis: Challenges in the Control and Eradication," in *Challenges in Infectious Diseases*, ed. I. W. Fong (New York: Springer, 2013), 247–264.

92. D. A. Henderson, "Eradication: Lessons from the Past," *Bulletin of the World Health Organization* 76, suppl. 2 (1998): 17–21.

93. M. J. Friedrich, "WHO Declares India Free of Yaws and Maternal and Neonatal Tetanus," *Journal of the American Medical Association* 316, no. 11 (2016): 1141.

94. M. Enserink, "What's Next for Disease Eradication?," *Science* 330, no. 6012 (2010): 1736–1739.

95. M. Morales, R. H. Tangermann, and S. G. Wassilak, "Progress toward Polio Eradication—Worldwide, 2015–2016," *Morbidity and Mortality Weekly Report* 65, no. 18 (2016): 470–473.

96. R. A. Harris, "A Thoroughly Modern Monarch: How the Queen Kept up with 70 Years of Constant Change," *The Sydney Morning Herald*, 3 June 2022.

97. L. O. Gostin, "Global Polio Eradication: Espionage, Disinformation, and the Politics of Vaccination," *The Milbank Quarterly* 92, no. 3 (2014): 413–417.

98. J. E. Hagan et al., "Progress toward Polio Eradication—Worldwide, 2014–2015," *Morbidity and Mortality Weekly Report* 64, no. 19 (2015): 527–531.

99. K. Esteves, "Safety of Oral Poliomyelitis Vaccine: Results of a WHO Enquiry," *Bulletin of the World Health Organization* 66, no. 6 (1988): 739–746.

100. "Poliomyelitis," *World Health Organization*, 22 July 2019, https://www.who.int/en/news-room/fact-sheets/detail/poliomyelitis (accessed 6 June 2022).

101. O. M. Kew et al., "Vaccine-Derived Polioviruses and the Endgame Strategy for Global Polio Eradication," *Annual Review of Microbiology* 59 (2005): 587–635.

102. R. Link-Gelles et al., "Public Health Response to a Case of Paralytic Poliomyelitis in an Unvaccinated Person and Detection of Poliovirus in Wastewater—New York, June–August 2022," *American Journal of Transplantation* 22, no. 10 (2022): 2470–2474.

103. D. R. Hopkins and E. Ruiz-Tiben, "Dracunculiasis (Guinea Worm Disease): Case Study of the Effort to Eradicate Guinea Worm," in *Water and Sanitation-Related Diseases and the Changing Environment*, ed. J.M.H. Selendy (Hoboken: Wiley-Blackwell, 2011), 283–290.

104. G. Biswas et al., "Dracunculiasis (Guinea Worm Disease): Eradication without a Drug or a Vaccine," *Philosophical Transactions of the Royal Society B: Biological Sciences* 368, no. 1623 (2013): 20120146.

105. S. Cairncross, E. I. Braide, and S. Z. Bugri, "Community Participation in the Eradication of Guinea Worm Disease," *Acta Tropica* 61 (1996): 121–136.

106. M. K. Kindhauser, *Communicable Diseases 2002: Global Defence against the Infectious Disease Threat* (Geneva: World Health Organization, 2003).

107. R. J. Smith? et al., "A Mathematical Model for the Eradication of Guinea Worm Disease," in *Understanding the Dynamics of Emerging and Re-Emerging Infectious Diseases using Mathematical Models*, ed. S. Mushayabasa and C. P. Bhunu (Kerala: Transworld Research, 2012), 133–156.

108. A. D. Kealey and R. J. Smith?, "Neglected Tropical Diseases: Infection, Modeling, and Control," *Journal of Health Care for the Poor and Underserved* 21 (2010): 53–69.

109. P. M. Wortley et al., "Healthcare Workers Who Elected Not to Receive Smallpox Vaccination," *American Journal of Preventive Medicine* 30, no. 3 (2006): 258–265.

110. F. Fenner et al., *Smallpox and Its Eradication*.

111. D. A. Koplow, *Smallpox: The Fight to Eradicate a Global Scourge* (Berkeley: University of California Press, 2003).

112. A. Wollenberg and R. Engler, "Smallpox, Vaccination and Adverse Reactions to Smallpox Vaccine," *Current Opinion in Allergy and Clinical Immunology* 4, no. 4 (2004): 271–275.

113. S. Riedel, "Smallpox and Biological Warfare: A Disease Revisited," *Baylor University Medical Center Proceedings* 18, no. 1 (2005): 13–20.

114. S. B. Lambert, "Disease Eradication Is Possible and Ethical," *The Lancet* 374 (2009): 1144.

115. A. Hochkirch et al., "License to Kill?—Disease Eradication Programs May Not Be in Line with the Convention on Biological Diversity," *Conservation Letters* 11 (2018): e12370.

116. B. Alyward et al., "When Is a Disease Eradicable? 100 Years of Lessons Learned," *American Journal of Health*, 90 (2000): 1515–1520.

117. P. P. Giorgi, S. Guy, and B. A. Hocking, "I Sing of Arms and the Doctor: What Role for Law When Biology Is Called to War?," in *The Nexus of Law and Biology*, ed. B. A. Hocking (London: Routledge, 2016), 53–74.

118. S. G. Stolberg and M. Peterson, "U.S. Orders Vast Supply of Vaccine for Smallpox," *The New York Times*, 29 November 2001.

119. N. Dewolf Smith, "Weaponized Soviet Smallpox—Where Is It Now?," *The Wall Street Journal*, 6 December 2002.

120. S. H. Harris, *Factories of Death: Japanese Biological Warfare 1932–45 and the American Cover-up* (London: Routledge, 1995).

121. K. Alibek and S. Handelman, *Biohazard: The Chilling True Story of the Largest Covert Biological Weapons Program in the World—Told from the Inside by the Man Who Ran It* (London: Delta, 2000).

122. G. A. Poland, R. B. Kennedy, and P. K. Tosh, "Prevention of Monkeypox with Vaccines: A Rapid Review," *The Lancet Infectious Diseases* 22, no. 12 (2022): e349–e358.

123. M. Wayne and B. Bolker, *Infectious Diseases: A Very Short Introduction* (Oxford: Oxford University Press, 2015).

124. B. J. Billioux et al., "Neurologic Complications of Smallpox and Monkeypox: A Review," *JAMA Neurology* 79, no. 11 (2022): 1180–1186.

125. D. Moschese et al., "Is Smallpox Vaccination Protective against Human Monkeypox?," *Journal of Medical Virology* 95, no. 1 (2022): e28077.

126. To Dr. Edward Jenner on His Discovery of the Small Pox Vaccine, Monticello, May 14, 1806, in *Letters of Thomas Jefferson 1743–1826*, http://www.let.rug.nl/usa/presidents/thomas-jefferson/letters-of-thomas-jefferson/jefl172.php (accessed 6 June 2022).

2 Tuberculosis

We mentioned in chapter 9 that most diseases are old. We weren't kidding: it's thought that tuberculosis (TB) originated more than 150 million years ago, during the Mesozoic Era.[1] Without any animal or insect reservoir, the geographic patterning of TB across now-disconnected regions suggests that it must have been present when they were last connected, back when most of the continents were one giant land mass known as Gondwanaland.[2] The breakup of this supercontinent 150 million years ago scattered humans across different continents, taking TB with them. The oldest definitive evidence of TB dates back 9,000 years, to a skeleton from Atlit Yam, a now-submerged Neolithic village off the coast of Israel.[3]

Unlike many other diseases we've covered, there was no animal origin. Human TB predates animal TB, including cattle, where it is known as bovine TB.[4] The disease is prevalent in a great many animals, both domestic and wild, in both herbivores (deer, sheep, goats, horses, pigs, camels, llamas, tapirs, elk, elephants, rhinoceroses, opossums, ground squirrels, otters, seals, and hares) and carnivores (dogs, cats, ferrets, foxes, badgers, rats, primates, moles, raccoons, coyotes, lions, tigers, leopards, and lynxes).[5] This thing is everywhere, but we were the first. (Hooray for us?)

TB DNA has been recovered from tissues of Egyptian mummies. There were TB hospitals in 1500 BCE,[6] and it's thought that the pharaoh Akhenaten (father of Tutankhamun) and his queen Nefertiti both died of it around 1330 BCE.[7] Egyptian mummies had skeletal deformities consistent with TB, with those deformities depicted in contemporary art, although no lesions are reported in the papyri.[8]

The first written account dates back 3,300 years to the *Rigveda*, an ancient Indian collection of Sanskrit hymns, where it was called "yaksma."[9] An Indian text from 600 BCE recommended the disease be countered with breast milk, various meats, alcohol, and rest, with another text recommending higher altitudes.[10] The latter wasn't so far off from modern methods, as we'll see.

Around 400 BCE, the classic Chinese medical text *Huangdi Neijing* called the disease "xulao bing" (weak consumptive disease), describing telltale symptoms such as coughing, fever, chest obstructions, and shortness of breath.[11] TB most commonly infects the respiratory tract, but it can also affect the gastrointestinal tract, bones, joints, nervous systems, lymph nodes, and other places.[12] The *Huangdi Neijing* referred to it as the "bad palace" (the palace being the chest) and noted the lack of any cure. The disease is also noted in the Bible in the books of Deuteronomy and Leviticus.[13]

In Ancient Greece, Isocrates was the first to postulate that TB might be an infectious disease. Hippocrates described it as a weakness of the lung, recognizing the predilection of the disease (as it was then) for those aged between 18 and 35.[14] He believed it to be hereditary, but Aristotle disagreed, believing it to be contagious.[15] The Greek physician Galen (who was Roman Emperor Marcus Aurelius's personal physician) recommended fresh air, milk, opium, bloodletting, and sea voyages as treatment, but the disease does not feature notably in the Roman histories.[16]

In a totally different part of the world, Peruvian mummies had TB 1,000 years ago.[17] In fact, so much genetic material was recovered from these mummies that scientists could reconstruct the TB genome.[18] However, infection of these mummies pre-dated Columbus. So how did they get it? One possibility, as noted above, is that the disease passed over land when all the continents were Gondwanaland. But there's another possibility, because the strain of TB found in Peru is related to that found in seals and sea lions.[19] It's thus thought that European TB may have travelled along trade routes and passed into domestic animals, then seals and sea lions, who carried it across the Atlantic to South America, where hunters contracted it.[20]

With such a widespread disease, myths were abundant. In twelfth-century Hungary, pagans believed that a dog-shaped demon occupied the body and began to eat the lungs.[21] A cough was a symbol of the dog barking, symbolizing the person's encroaching death as the dog got closer to its objective. Among the Akan tribe in Ghana, there was a belief that TB could arise from ancestral punishment due to lack of care provided to family members who had suffered and died from TB; others believed that tuberculosis was a spiritual disease and therefore did not need any medical attention.[22]

In Europe during the Middle Ages and the Renaissance, TB slowly replaced leprosy as the disease of the poor.[23] In 1546, the Italian physician Girolamo Fracastoro was the first person to propose that it was transmitted by an invisible virus, suggesting that it was passed by direct contact or bodily fluids and could survive on clothes.[24] Fracastoro invented the word "fomes" to describe the non-living surfaces that retain germs, from which we get "fomites" (a term that became better known when COVID-19 first arrived and surfaces that might carry the infection had to be cleaned to a high standard). In 1689, Richard Morton was the first to establish that tuberculosis is always associated with the tubercles (nodules) that form in different parts of the body.[25]

TB was called "consumption" during the seventeenth and eighteenth centuries and was nicknamed the "robber of youth" for its high mortality among people in the prime of their life.[26] Case numbers rose as a large-scale epidemic began to sweep across Europe. By the late seventeenth century, the London Bills of Mortality reported that consumption was responsible for a quarter of all deaths in the city.[27] The Industrial Revolution was a driving factor, with incidence rising as field workers moved to cities, which became denser and in parts more squalid, thus facilitating the spread of the disease. Industrialization, urbanization, and TB became so inextricably linked that they were seen as necessary steps on a country's path to modernity.[28] Epidemics in Europe and North America during the eighteenth and nineteenth centuries led to a different nickname for the disease: "Captain Among These Men of Death."[29] The disease was the nineteenth century's greatest killer.[30]

Society responded by romanticizing the disease, with wan and pallid faces considered attractive. This appearance gave it yet another nickname: the White Plague. Due to the epidemic coinciding with the surge in Romanticism, which stressed feeling over reason, it was often referred to as "the romantic disease," with sufferers thought to achieve heightened sensitivity.[31] Chopin's lover called him her "poor melancholy angel," writing "Chopin coughs with infinite grace," while Lord Byron expressed a wish to die of consumption, because it would mean all the ladies would remark how interesting he would look in death.[32] When a statue was commissioned of John Harvard (who lent his name to the famous university) in 1884, no pictures of the man existed, but it was recorded that he died aged 30 of consumption,[33] so it was assumed that his face would have been delicate and his expression sensitive.[34] Non-afflicted upper-class women would purposefully pale their skin to achieve the consumptive appearance.[35]

Down in the lower classes, the poor fared less elegantly. Quarantine, prohibitions against spitting, and strict guidelines on caring for children and infants were routinely ignored, leading politicians to blame the poor for their own plight.[36]

Les Misérables was just one of the novels of the time to express the idealized public perceptions of TB.[37] Likewise, Puccini's opera *La Bohème* (retold more recently as the musical and film *Moulin Rouge*) dwells on both the tragedy and the romanticism of TB.[38] The slow progress allowed for a good death, as sufferers could put their affairs in order.[39] The appeal of the disease's redemptive-spiritual aspects remained even after medical breakthroughs in understanding.[40]

Another moniker for TB was "the king's evil," because of belief that a royal touch could cure it.[41] Royals were believed to be divine, with the power to cure diseases and conditions. On Easter 1608, King Henry IV of France performed the royal touch on 1,250 infected people in a single event.[42] This was initially done informally, during the king's walkabouts, but by the time of King Louis XIV of France, with the epidemic sweeping the nation, placards indicated the days and times the king was available for royal touches, with charitable donations collected.[43]

In England, the process was formal, and the afflicted were gifted a coin, pressed against their neck. Parish records from Oxfordshire include baptisms, marriages, deaths, and details of those eligible for the royal touch.[44] In 1712, Queen Anne was the last English monarch to use this practice, a young Samuel Johnson being among those she touched.[45] George I put a stop to it in 1714, but French monarchs continued it until 1825.[46]

TB as an infectious agent caused by "wonderfully minute living creatures" was conjectured in 1720 by English physician Benjamin Marten.[47] This theory was roundly rejected by the medical community and remained so for another 162 years. Modern understanding of the disease began with French physician René Laennec's 1819 treatise on the subject.[48] Laennec is best known for inventing the stethoscope, but he unified the different manifestations of TB, whether pulmonary or extrapulmonary, describing signs of the disease using terminology we still use today. Laennec had vast experience due to the epidemic sweeping across Europe in this time, with death rates in London, Stockholm, and Hamburg approaching 1.25% of all deaths. Laennec himself died of the disease at 45 after studying the infection in contagious patients and infected bodies.[49] (His nephew diagnosed him with the disease using Laennec's own stethoscope.)[50] Laennec is remembered today as France's greatest physician.

The infectious nature of the disease was demonstrated in 1865 by Jean-Antoine Villemin, a French military surgeon, after noticing different effects on soldiers stationed in barracks compared to those in the field.[51] He also observed that healthy new recruits from the country became infected some months after joining the military.[52] He performed experiments on rabbits to prove the infection.[53] Rabbits are generally resistant to TB, so he got lucky; he might have had even more dramatic results if he'd used guinea pigs, which are far more susceptible to it.[54]

Legions of famous people died from TB. St Francis of Assisi died of it in 1226 aged 44.[55] Jane Austen died from TB,[56] as did Louis Braille, Anton Chekhov, Franz Kafka, George Orwell, John Keats, and the Brontë sisters. Eleanor Roosevelt died of complications from TB she had as a child.[57] Even my own grandmother died of it, in the 1980s. TB has killed a whopping *one billion* people in the past 200 years.[58] Consumption was the most common killer of colonial American adults, accounting for more than a quarter of all deaths in New York City between 1810 and 1815, for example.

In the eighteenth and nineteenth centuries, treatment involved puncturing or collapsing the lungs in the hopes of sterilizing the sputum via cavity closure. This was based on a much older example: a TB patient improved in 1696 after a sword wound, leading to pulmonary-collapse therapy as a treatment in order to "rest" diseased lungs by puncturing them.[59]

A less invasive remedy than puncturing lungs arrived in the form of sanatoriums,[60] specialized hospitals for the treatment of specific diseases. Harriet Ryan Albee had opened the Channing Home in the basement of a Boston church in 1857.[61] However, the concept took off thanks to Hermann Brehmer, a botany student who had suffered from TB himself but who had healed after travelling to the Himalayas.[62] Brehmer opened his *Heilenstat* in Göbersdorf, Poland, in 1859, which became the model for sanatoriums ever since.[63] Brehmer believed that TB arose from the difficulty of the heart to irrigate the lungs and thus believed that regions well above sea level, with lower atmospheric pressure, would help the heart function more effectively; Göbersdorf was 650 metres above sea level.[64]

Sanitoriums for the middle and upper classes offered excellent care and constant medical attention, while the poor were pressured to enter sanitoriums that resembled prisons. A later five-year study compared patients treated at home to those treated in sanitoriums: death rates among patients with minimal disease was 14% in sanitoriums versus 38% at home, whereas those with advanced disease died at rates of 61% in sanitoriums versus 81% at home.[65] Sanatoriums became inextricably linked with TB in popular literature.[66]

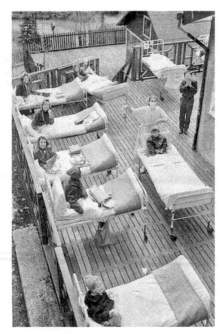

Figure 2.1. TB patients at the outdoor "Fresh Air School" in Montréal, 1939.

Source: Photograph by Ted Hill and made available by John E. Hill.

TB began to decline in the mid-nineteenth century, but the reasons for this remain elusive. Partial explanations include improving sanitation and living conditions in high-income countries, herd immunity, and improved nutrition.[67] Concurrently, the disease shifted from one in young people to one in the elderly, as a legacy of their high infection rates when they were young.[68] Improved building ventilations in the nineteenth and twentieth centuries also contributed to the decline of tuberculosis and several other airborne diseases, such as smallpox and influenza, in high-income countries. However, such practices have waned in more recent years as the focus has switched to energy-efficient buildings rather than well-ventilated ones.[69] Low-tech solutions to age-old problems such as ventilated buildings for TB have been applied in low- and middle-income countries where costs of mechanical ventilators for individual patients are prohibitive.[70]

Prussian physician Robert Koch (who had previously elucidated the life cycle of anthrax and invented the Petri dish) isolated the causative bacillus in 1882, confirming Marten's theory about tiny creatures causing disease and essentially founding the field of bacteriology.[71] This discovery electrified the medical community and earned Koch the Nobel Prize in Medicine in 1905.[72] The World Health Organization chose March 24 as World Tuberculosis Day in commemoration of the date of Koch's announcement of his finding.[73]

From this discovery of the cause of TB, Koch isolated a substance that could be injected; he even injected himself with concentrated tuberculin and observed an unusually violent attack of fever and rise in body temperature up to 39.6°C.[74] Although smallpox vaccination had been underway for almost a century, vaccination as a concept was still relatively new; the second human vaccine, a rabies vaccine developed by Louis Pasteur, was still a few years away.[75] While Koch's "treatment" was quickly dismissed as ineffective (tuberculin killed more people than it helped), this breakthrough was developed into a diagnostic test, which was soon being used to identify the disease in cattle.[76] Koch laid down a series of conditions known as the Koch postulates that must be satisfied before it could be accepted that particular bacteria caused specific diseases.[77]

Physician Edward Livingston Trudeau, who had suffered from TB himself, established the Adirondack Sanatorium in 1885. Author Robert Louis Stevenson was an early patient, and his fame helped popularize it. Trudeau wrote: "My faith in the possibilities of chemotherapy* for tuberculosis is based simply on what Ehrlich has demonstrated as possible in syphilis—namely, that a chemical compound could be discovered which killed the germ without injuring the cell [...] I see no reason why what has been accomplished in the treatment of syphilis should not be attained in tuberculosis."[78]

One of the first medical experts to have a radio program was American physician Hermann Biggs, who was general medical officer of the New York City Metropolitan Board of Health, the first modern public-health authority in the United States.[79] In 1889, Biggs required doctors to report all cases of TB.[80] This was resisted by both the public and the medical profession, but Koch noted it as a practical public-health tool.[81] Notifiable diseases are a method we still use today in order to track infections.

The worldwide death rate due to TB at the end of the nineteenth century was 7 million people per year, with 50 million openly infected.[82] London and New York were the worst-hit cities.[83] Concerns about TB in the United States led to public spitting being prohibited, except into spittoons.[84] At the turn of the twentieth century, TB was one of the U.K.'s most urgent problems. A royal commission was set up in 1901 to study animal and human TB.[85] By 1919, this commission had evolved into the U.K.'s Medical Research Council. Following New York's example, TB was made a notifiable disease in Great Britain.

A skin test was developed in 1907 by Clemens von Pirquet, one of Vienna's leading paediatricians. Von Pirquet coined the terms "allergy," "allergen," and "latent," the latter in the context of TB, and was the person who first described boosters for the immune system.[86] He built off Koch's work and found that exposing a small amount of diluted tuberculin intracutaneously would detect latent TB in children.[87]

Therapeutic pneumothorax (lung collapsing) saw a resurgence in the early twentieth century, although there were no controlled studies of its efficacy, not least because such studies would have been difficult to construct.[88] By 1955, collapse therapy had been replaced by resection surgery (removing part or all the diseased tissue), and by 1958 resection surgery had been supplanted by chemotherapy.[89]

---

* "Chemotherapy" is used here to refer to any therapy involving chemicals, rather than the exclusively cancer-based treatment that the term is used for today.

Chest radiographs were used by both the Germans and the Allies during the First World War to screen recruits for TB. The American Red Cross sponsored a trip by New York's Hermann Biggs to France in 1916–1917 to assess the state of TB, where he found that it was a problem of "stupendous magnitude," with around half a million cases and no facilities to care for them.[90] As a result, there was a U.S.–French partnership campaign to bring public-health measures and education about TB to France that led to a significant post-war decline in cases.[91]

After so many deaths and so much time, a vaccine was developed by Albert Calmette, one of the founding directors of the Pasteur Institute (and the first person to develop an antivenom for snake bites).[92] In 1921, Calmette and his assistant Camille Guérin (a veterinarian) attenuated *M. bovis* for use as a vaccine, giving it first to an infant born of a mother dying of pulmonary TB.[93] The baby survived and did not develop the disease, so more than 100,000 children were immunized over the next seven years, including Calmette's.[94] The vaccine was named the Bacille Calmette–Guérin (BCG) vaccine. The vaccine suffered a setback in 1930 when 73 vaccinated German children developed tuberculosis and died due to contamination of some batches.[95] The vaccine was popular in Europe but was not used in Britain until 1950 and was never used on a large scale in the United States.[96]

In Indigenous American populations of the 1930s, the disease was so widespread that approximately 75% of the native population was infected. In Saskatchewan, 29% of all First Nations, Métis, and Inuit deaths were from TB. And in what is now Arizona and Northern Mexico, a shocking 100% of the Akimel O'odham people over the age of 20 were infected with the disease.[97]

TB was *the* major health disaster of the Second World War, with malnutrition, overcrowding, and disruption of medical services driving factors in the spread of the disease.[98] In Nazi-occupied Poland, more than 30,000 TB-infected patients were executed.[99] TB was one of the prevailing diseases in concentration camps, due to filthy living conditions and severe malnutrition.[100] Food shortages in cities contributed to the spread, while TB strains increased in malignancy by the end of the war.[101]

Treatment with the antibiotic streptomycin (see chapter 10) was developed in 1944.[102] Furthermore, the latently infected could be treated, rather than just those with symptoms.[103] Following the Second World War, a widespread testing and treatment program began in Poland, which spread to other European countries (and Ecuador); 30 million people were tested and 14 million vaccinated.[104] This was the first disease-control program undertaken by the newly formed World Health Organization in 1950.[105] The key breakthrough came in 1952 with the development of isoniazid, an orally administered treatment, while rifampin was developed in the 1970s and hastened recovery times.[106]

The 1956 Madras Experiment in India found no noticeable differences in recovery rates between patients in sanatoriums versus at home. This discovery, along with vaccination, led to the closure of sanatoriums as a treatment for TB.[107] The Madras Experiment demonstrated that large-scale randomized controlled trials could be undertaken in difficult settings, proving to be one of the most cost-effective studies ever conducted.[108]

Mortality declined throughout the second half of the twentieth century, but to what extent this was due to vaccination and treatment is questionable.

Instead, as with improving numbers in the nineteenth century, better hygiene, nutrition, and general standards of living had an outsized effect on disease reduction.[109] British epidemiologist Thomas McKeown, considered the father of social medicine, advocated that drugs and vaccines only go so far and that diseases of poverty will not be controlled until improvements are made in air quality, water, sanitation, housing, education, safety, and justice.[110]

Like all diseases, society's treatment of those afflicted with TB varies enormously, depending on who has power. In Canada, surgical resection of TB was carried out in Indigenous patients during the 1950s and 1960s, long after the process had been abandoned in non-Indigenous populations.[111] Increased pressure on wages by IMF loans to post-communist Eastern Europe were strongly associated with a rise in TB cases in the 1990s.[112]

Drug-resistant TB had been noticed as early as 1948 but grew throughout the second half of the twentieth century.[113] TB has a low natural mutation rate, but evolutionary pressure from drugs sped it up. Cases in Britain fell throughout most of the twentieth century but rose towards the end and plateaued thereafter.[114] Resistance to a single drug was bad enough, but the real danger came from multi-drug resistance, when TB becomes resistant to at least two of the drugs, making it almost impossible to treat.[115] Elimination of public-health facilities in New York was partially responsible for a resurgence there in the 1980s, with 52,000 TB cases in New York City, of which almost a quarter were multi-drug resistant.[116]

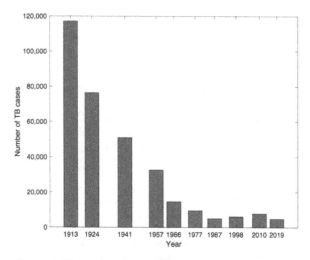

Figure 2.2. TB cases in England and Wales.
Source: Public Health England, *Tuberculosis (TB): Annual Notification Data 1913 Onwards*, 23 October 2020.

There's another factor in play, which is HIV. Co-infection is common, with the weaker immune systems of HIV patients making them particularly susceptible to TB. This is bad enough for the wild-type strain of TB, but HIV in combination with multi-drug-resistant TB or extensively drug-resistant TB is especially dangerous.[117]

In 1993, the World Health Organization declared TB to be a public-health emergency, ending a long period of global neglect.[118] In 1994, they proposed Directly Observed Treatment, Short course (DOTS) to verify that treatment was actually taken. A problem with TB treatment is that if the course of treatment is not completed, the effect is essentially zero. It is crucial to ensure treatment is actually administered to completion, thus requiring treatment to occur in medical facilities under observation, rather than at home.[119] In Australia, TB was being brought into the north by Torres Strait Islanders (who have free right of travel between Australia and Papua New Guinea, provided the intended travel is for traditional purposes), so the Australian government funded an expansion of DOTS in Papua New Guinea, which was a cost-effective way of controlling the disease in both countries.[120] Individuals with TB were originally eligible to receive treatment in Australian facilities even if they were not Australian residents; this eligibility was later removed, except in the case of triage, as healthcare was not considered a traditional activity.[121]

In 2017, two billion people were infected with TB worldwide, with 10.4 million new cases per year.[122] The European and North American decline has continued, but in other places, especially where fuelled by HIV, the epidemic continues. TB has evolved into a disease that we treat, much more than one we vaccinate against. Vaccination occurs primarily in newborns, while TB-control programs emphasize treatment of latently infected individuals.[123]

Today, despite being curable and preventable, TB remains the second leading cause of death from an infectious disease worldwide.[124] Only COVID-19 is deadlier.

Table 2.1. Timeline of tuberculosis

150000000 BCE	Origins
9000 BCE	Oldest known TB skeleton
1330 BCE	Queen Nefertiti dies
1300 BCE	First written account
1266 CE	Death of St Francis of Assisi
1546 CE	Viral form proposed
1720 CE	Germ theory conjectured
1857 CE	First sanatorium opens
1882 CE	Bacillus isolated
1921 CE	BCG vaccine developed
1944 CE	Antibiotic treatment developed
1993 CE	TB declared a world health emergency
2017 CE	Two billion infected worldwide

Source: Summary of this chapter.

Notes

1. I. Barberis et al., "The History of Tuberculosis: From the First Historical Records to the Isolation of Koch's Bacillus," *Journal of Preventive Medicine and Hygiene* 58, no. 1 (2017): E9–E12.

2. J. Hayman, "Mycobacterium ulcerans: An Infection from Jurassic Time?," *The Lancet* 324, no. 8410 (1984): 1015–1016.

3. M. Spigelman et al., "Evolutionary Changes in the Genome of Mycobacterium Tuberculosis and the Human Genome from 9000 Years BP until Modern Times," *Tuberculosis* 95 (2015): S145–S149.

4. S. Gagneux, "Host–Pathogen Coevolution in Human Tuberculosis," *Philosophical Transactions of the Royal Society B: Biological Sciences* 367, no. 1590 (2012): 850–859.

5. C. O. Thoen, P. A. LoBue, and D. A. Enarson, "Tuberculosis in Animals and Humans: An Introduction," in *Zoonotic Tuberculosis: Mycobacterium bovis and other Pathogenic Mycobacteria*, ed. C. Thoen, J. H. Steele, and J. B. Kaneene (Hoboken: Wiley-Blackwell, 2014), 3–7.

6. M. M. Monir, *Tuberculosis* (Berlin: Springer Verlag, 2004).

7. C. Morazzoni and M. DePaschale, "The History of Tuberculosis: From Mummies to Multidrug Resistance across the Royal Touch," *Microbiologia Medica* 31, no. 2 (2016): 5782.

8. A. J. E. Cave, "The Evidence for the Incidence of Tuberculosis in Ancient Egypt," *British Journal of Tuberculosis* 33 (1939): 142–152.

9. S. P. Tripathy et al., "History of Tuberculosis," *National Medicos Organisation Journal* 12, no. 1 (2018): 14–18.

10. P. R. Bapat et al., "Prevalence of Zoonotic Tuberculosis and Associated Risk Factors in Central Indian Populations," *Journal of Epidemiology and Global Health* 7, no. 4 (2017): 277–283.

11. N. Mishra, S. Kant, and K. Srivastava, "Landmarks in Tuberculosis," *National Medicos Organisation Journal* 12, no. 1 (2018): 26–28.

12. B. Varghese et al., "Impact of Mycobacterium Tuberculosis Complex Lineages as a Determinant of Disease Phenotypes from an Immigrant Rich Moderate Tuberculosis Burden Country," *Respiratory Research* 19, no. 1 (2018): 1–9.

13. V. S. Daniel and T. M. Daniel, "Old Testament Biblical References to Tuberculosis," *Clinical Infectious Diseases* 29, no. 6 (1999): 1557–1558.

14. V. N. Houk, "Spread of Tuberculosis via Recirculated Air in a Naval Vessel: The Byrd Study," *Annals of the New York Academy of Sciences* 353, no. 1 (1980): 10–24.

15. M. E. Molyneux, "Straight and Crooked Thinking about Tuberculosis," *South African Medical Journal* 62, no. 21 (1982): 34–35.

16. G. P. Williams, "A Talmudic Perspective on the Old Testament Diseases, Physicians and Remedies" (doctoral thesis, University of South Africa, 2009).

17. W. L. Salo et al., "Identification of Mycobacterium Tuberculosis DNA in a Pre-Columbian Peruvian Mummy," *Proceedings of the National Academy of Sciences* 91, no. 6 (1994): 2091–2094.

18. L. A. Arriola, A. Cooper, and L. S. Weyrich, "Palaeomicrobiology: Application of Ancient DNA Sequencing to Better Understand Bacterial Genome Evolution and Adaptation," *Frontiers in Ecology and Evolution* 8 (2020): 40.

19. L. Zmak et al., "From Peruvian Mummies to Living Humans: First Case of Pulmonary Tuberculosis Caused by Mycobacterium pinnipedii," *The International Journal of Tuberculosis and Lung Disease* 23, no. 12 (2019): 1283–1285.

20. A. Kiers et al., "Transmission of Mycobacterium pinnipedii to Humans in a Zoo with Marine Mammals," *The International Journal of Tuberculosis and Lung Disease* 12, no. 12 (2008): 1469–1473.

21. I. A. Hussein, "Statistical Analysis of Socio-Economic and Cultural Correlates of Lung Tuberculosis: A Case Study of Wad Medani Teaching Hospital, Gezira State, Sudan" (doctoral dissertation, University of Gezira, 2018).

22. R. Cofie and A. Liu, "Knowledge, Myths and Misconceptions of Ghanaians about Tuberculosis," *International Journal of Advanced Physiology and Allied Sciences* 2, no. 1 (2014): 24–30.

23. S. R. Wood, "A Contribution to the History of Tuberculosis and Leprosy in 19th Century Norway," *Journal of the Royal Society of Medicine* 84, no. 7 (1991): 428–430.

24. H. K. Jabr, "Tuberculosis as a Re-Emerging Disease" (master's thesis, Cairo University, 2012).

25. J. A. Silverman, "Richard Morton, 1637–1698 Limner of Anorexia Nervosa: His Life and Times: A Tercentenary Essay," *Journal of the American Medical Association* 250, no. 20 (1983): 2830–2382.

26. Y. Agarwal et al., "The Tuberculosis Timeline: Of White Plague, a Birthday Present, and Vignettes of Myriad Hues," *Astrocyte* 4, no. 1 (2017): 7–26.

27. M. K. Matossian, "Death in London, 1750–1909. *The Journal of Interdisciplinary History* 16, no. 2 (1985):183–197, 1985.

28. C. W McMillen, *Pandemics: A Very Short Introduction* (Oxford: Oxford University Press, 2016).

29. A. Y. Ayinla, W. A. Othman, and M. Rabiu, "A Mathematical Model of the Tuberculosis Epidemic," *Acta Biotheoretica* 69, no. 3 (2021): 225–255.

30. C. W McMillen, *Pandemics*.

31. S. Sontag, *Illness as Metaphor* (New York: Farrar, 1978).

32. C. F. Giuliano, "Gulnare/Kaled's 'Untold' Feminization of Byron's Oriental Tales," *Studies in English Literature, 1500–1900* 33, no. 4 (1993): 785–807.

33. E. R. Grigg, "The Arcana of Tuberculosis: With a Brief Epidemiologic History of the Disease in the USA Part III," *American Review of Tuberculosis and Pulmonary Diseases* 78, no. 3 (1958): 426–453.

34. M. Richman, "The Man Who Made John Harvard," *Harvard Magazine* 80 (1977): 46–51.

35. Y. Agarwal et al., "The Tuberculosis Timeline: Of White Plague, a Birthday Present, and Vignettes of Myriad Hues".

36. D. Armus, *The Ailing City: Health, Tuberculosis, and Culture in Buenos Aires, 1870–1950* (Durham: Duke University Press, 2011).

37. M. A. Schwartz, "Tuberculosis—A Journey across Time," *Tuberculosis* 1, no. 4 (2009).

38. F. Cantini and D. Goletti, "Biologics and Tuberculosis Risk: The Rise and Fall of an Old Disease and Its New Resurgence," *The Journal of Rheumatology* 91 (2014): 1–3.

39. P. Bourdelais, *Epidemics Laid Low: A History of What Happened in Rich Countries* (Baltimore: Johns Hopkins University Press, 2006).

40. D. S. Barnes, *The Making of a Social Disease: Tuberculosis in Nineteenth-Century France* (Berkeley: University of California Press, 1995).

41. I. Barberis et al., "The History of Tuberculosis: From the First Historical Records to the Isolation of Koch's Bacillus".

42. J. C. Cataño and J. Robledo, "Tuberculous Lymphadenitis and Parotitis," in *Tuberculosis and Nontuberculous Mycobacterial Infections* ed. D. Schlossberg (Washington, DC: American Society for Microbiology, 2017), 343–354.

43. C. Morazzoni and M. DePaschale, "The History of Tuberculosis: From Mummies to Multidrug Resistance across the Royal Touch".

44. R. C. Maulitz and S. R. Maulitz, "The King's Evil in Oxfordshire," *Medical History* 17, no. 1 (1973): 87–89.

45. I. Barberis et al., "The History of Tuberculosis: From the First Historical Records to the Isolation of Koch's Bacillus".

46. J. Frith, "History of Tuberculosis Part 1—Pthisis, Consumption and the White Plague," *Journal of Military and Veterans' Health* 22, no. 2 (2014): 29–35.

47. R. N. Doetsch, "Benjamin Marten and His 'New Theory of Consumptions,'" *Microbiological Reviews* 42, no. 3 (1978): 521–528.

48. J. Frith, "History of Tuberculosis Part 1—Pthisis, Consumption and the White Plague".

49. R. M. Wishnow and J. L. Steinfeld, "The Conquest of the Major Infectious Diseases in the United States: A Bicentennial Retrospect," *Annual Review of Microbiology* 30, no. 1 (1976): 427–450.

50. A. Roguin, "Rene Theophile Hyacinthe Laënnec (1781–1826): The Man behind the Stethoscope," *Clinical Medicine & Research* 4, no. 3 (2006): 230–235.

51. T. M. Daniel, "Jean-Antoine Villemin and the Infectious Nature of Tuberculosis," *The International Journal of Tuberculosis and Lung Disease* 19, no. 3 (2015): 267–268.

52. J. F. Murray, "History of Tuberculosis and of Warfare," in *Tuberculosis and War*, ed. J. F. Murray and R. Loddenkemper (Basel: Karger, 2018), 2–19.

53. A. Contrepois and A. M. Moulin, "Early History of Animal Models of Infection," in *Handbook of Animal Models of Infection*, ed. O. Zak and M. A. Sande (London: Academic Press, 1999), 3–8.

54. T. M. Daniel, "The History of Tuberculosis," *Respiratory Medicine* 100 (2006): 1862–1870.

55. H. Viviers, "The Second Christ, Saint Francis of Assisi and Ecological Consciousness," *Verbum et Ecclesia* 35, no. 1 (2014): 1–9.

56. G. A. Wilson, "An Historical Ophthalmic Study of Jane Austen," *British Journal of Ophthalmology* 96, no. 11 (2012): 1365–1367.

57. B. Lerner, "Revisiting the Death of Eleanor Roosevelt: Was the Diagnosis of Tuberculosis Missed?," *The International Journal of Tuberculosis and Lung Disease* 5, no. 12 (2001): 1080–1085.

58. N. M. Parrish, J. D. Dick, and W. R. Bishai, "Mechanisms of Latency in Mycobacterium Tuberculosis," *Trends in Microbiology* 6, no. 3 (1998): 107–112.

59. P. Humphreys, "The Magic Mountain—A Time Capsule of Tuberculosis Treatment in the early Twentieth Century," *Canadian Bulletin of Medical History* 6, no. 2 (1989): 147–163.

60. J. F. Murray, D. E. Schraufnagel, and P. C. Hopewell, "Treatment of Tuberculosis. A Historical Perspective," *Annals of the American Thoracic Society* 12, no. 12 (2015): 1749–1759.

61. T. M. Daniel, *Times and Tides of Tuberculosis: Perceptions Revealed in Literature, Keats to Sontag* (McKinleyville: Fithian Press, 2013).

62. I. Barberis et al., "The History of Tuberculosis: From the First Historical Records to the Isolation of Koch's Bacillus," Journal of Preventive Medicine and Hygiene 58, no. 1 (2017): E9–E12.

63. I. Barberis et al., "Tuberculosis from the First Ancient Historical Records," *Breminate*, 18 November 2021.

64. A. Jüttemann, "History of the Prussian Tuberculosis Sanatorium Movement, 1863–1934," *Acta Medicorum Polonorum* 5, no. 1 (2015): 5–14.

65. G. Lissant Cox, "Sanatorium Treatment Contrasted with Home Treatment," *British Journal of Tuberculosis* 17, no. 1 (1923): 27–30.

66. T. Mann, *Der Zauberberg* ("The Magic Mountain") (Berlin: Fischer Verlag, 1923).

67. K. F. Ortblad et al., "Stopping Tuberculosis: A Biosocial Model for Sustainable Development," *The Lancet* 386, no. 10010 (2015): 2354–2362.

68. K. F. Andvord, "What Can We Learn by Following the Development of Tuberculosis from One Generation to Another?," *International Journal of Tuberculosis Lung Disease* 6 (2002): 562–568.

69. S. Zhang, "We're Just Rediscovering a 19th-Century Pandemic Strategy," *The Atlantic*, 22 February 2021.

70. J. R. Minkel, "A Breath of Fresh Air: To Fight Tuberculosis, Open a Window," *Scientific American*, 26 February 2007.

71. S. M. Blevins and M. S. Bronze, "Robert Koch and the 'Golden Age' of Bacteriology," *International Journal of Infectious Diseases* 14, no. 9 (2010): e744–751.

72. A. Grzybowski and K. Pietrzak, "Robert Koch (1843–1910) and Dermatology on His 171st Birthday," *Clinics in Dermatology* 32, no. 3 (2014): 448–450.

73. T. Ulrichs, "The Berlin Declaration on Tuberculosis and Its Consequences for TB Research and Control in the WHO-Euro Region," *European Journal of Microbiology and Immunology* 2, no. 4 (2012): 261–263.

74. M. Martini, G. Besozzi, and I. Barberis, "The Never-Ending Story of the Fight against Tuberculosis: From Koch's Bacillus to Global Control Programs," *Journal of Preventive Medicine and Hygiene* 59, no. 3 (2018): E241–E247.

75. D. J. Hicks, A. R. Fooks, and N. Johnson, "Developments in Rabies Vaccines," *Clinical & Experimental Immunology* 169, no. 3 (2012): 199–204.

76. C. Gradmann, "Robert Koch and the Pressures of Scientific Research: Tuberculosis and Tuberculin," *Medical History* 45, no. 1 (2001): 1–32.

77. T. M. Rivers, "Viruses and Koch's Postulates," *Journal of Bacteriology* 33, no. 1 (1937): 1–12.

78. J. Frith, "History of Tuberculosis. Part 2—The Sanatoria and the Discoveries of the Tubercle Bacillus," *Journal of Military and Veterans Health* 22, no. 2 (2014): 36–41.

79. C.-E. A. Winslow, "The Contribution of Hermann Biggs to Public Health," *American Review of Tuberculosis* 20, no. 1 (1929): 1–28.

80. T. R. Frieden, B. H. Lerner, and B. R. Rutherford, "Lessons from the 1800s: Tuberculosis Control in the New Millennium," *The Lancet* 355, no. 9209 (2000): 1088–1092.

81. C.-E.A. Winslow, *The Life of Hermann M. Biggs, M.D., D.Sc., LL.D. Physician and Statesman of the Public Health* (Philadelphia: Lea & Feiberger, 1929).

82. R. Frank, *The Forgotten Plague: How the Battle against Tuberculosis Was Won—And Lost* (Boston: Little, Brown and Company, 1993).

83. P. Brown, "A Disease That Is Alive and Kicking," *World Health* 46, no. 4 (1993): 4–5.

84. J. E. Abrams, "'Spitting Is Dangerous, Indecent, and against the Law!' Legislating Health Behavior during the American Tuberculosis Crusade," *Journal of the History of Medicine and Allied Sciences* 68, no. 3 (2013): 416–450.

85. J. S. Fowler, "A Résumé of the Report of the Royal Commission on Human and Bovine Tuberculosis," *Edinburgh Medical Journal* 23, no. 3 (1908): 232–236.

86. E. L. Becker, "Elements of the History, of Our Present Concepts of Anaphylaxis, Hay Fever and Asthma," *Clinical and Experimental Allergy* 29 (1999): 875–895.

87. D. E. Snider, "The Tuberculin Skin Test," *American Review of Respiratory Disease* 125, 3P2 (1982): 108–118.

88. N. Hansson and I. J. Polianski, "Therapeutic Pneumothorax and the Nobel Prize," *The Annals of Thoracic Surgery* 100, no. 2 (2015): 761–765.

89. W. S. Conklin, "Surgical Trends in Pulmonary Tuberculosis," *Diseases of the Chest* 27, no. 2 (1955): 147–164.

90. H. Biggs, "Tuberculosis in France," *American Journal of Public Health* 7, no. 7 (1917): 606–611.

91. J. F. Murray, "Tuberculosis and World War I," *American Journal of Respiratory and Critical Care Medicine* 192, no. 4 (2015): 411–414.

92. B. J. Hawgood, "Albert Calmette (1863–1933) and Camille Guerin (1872–1961): The C and G of BCG Vaccine," *Journal of Medical Biography* 15, no. 3 (2007): 139–146.

93. S. Charoenlap, K. Piromsopa, and C. Charoenlap, "Potential Role of Bacillus Calmette-Guérin (BCG) Vaccination in COVID-19 Pandemic Mortality: Epidemiological and Immunological Aspects," *Asian Pacific Journal of Allergy and Immunology* 38, no. 3 (2020): 150–161.

94. M. Clark and D. W. Cameron, "The Benefits and Risks of Bacille Calmette-Guérin Vaccination among Infants at High Risk for Both Tuberculosis and Severe Combined Immunodeficiency: Assessment by Markov Model," *BMC Pediatrics* 6, no. 1 (2006): 1–2.

95. A. Sakula, "BCG: Who Were Calmette and Guérin?," *Thorax* 38, no. 11 (1983): 806–812.

96. L. Bryder, "'We Shall Not Find Salvation in Inoculation': BCG Vaccination in Scandinavia, Britain and the USA, 1921–1960," *Social Science & Medicine* 49, no. 9 (1999): 1157–1167.

97. C. W. McMillen, *Pandemics*.

98. R. Loddenkemper and J. F. Murray, *Tuberculosis and War: Lessons Learned from World War II* (Basel: Karger, 2018).

99. A. Finley-Croswhite and A. Munzer, "Nazi Medicine, Tuberculosis, and Genocide," in *Tuberculosis and War*, ed. R. Loddenkemper and J. F. Murray (Basel: Karger, 2018), 44–62.

100. R. Loddenkemper and N. Konietzko, "Tuberculosis in Germany before, during and after World War II," in *Tuberculosis and War*, ed. R. Loddenkemper and J. F. Murray (Basel: Karger, 2018), 64–85.

101. J. Grosset and A. Trébucq, "Tuberculosis in France before, during, and after World War II," in *Tuberculosis and War*, ed. R. Loddenkemper and J. F. Murray (Basel: Karger, 2018), 116–123.

102. C. Hinshaw, W. H. Feldman, and K. H. Pfuetze, "Treatment of Tuberculosis with Streptomycin: A Summary of Observations on One Hundred Cases," *Journal of the American Medical Association* 132, no. 13 (1946): 778–782.

103. D. Shingadia and V. Novelli, "Diagnosis and Treatment of Tuberculosis in Children," *The Lancet Infectious Diseases* 3, no. 10 (2003): 624–632.

104. "Mass BCG Vaccination Campaigns: 1948–1951," *World Health Organization*, https://apps.who.int/iris/handle/10665/62743 (accessed 7 June 2022).

105. *The First Ten Years of the World Health Organization* (Geneva: World Health Organization, 1958).

106. R. Singh, P. Kumar, and K. Tahlan, "Drugs against Mycobacterium Tuberculosis," in *Drug Discovery Targeting Drug-Resistant Bacteria*, ed. P. Kesharwani, S. Chopra, and A. Dasgupta (London: Academic Press, 2020), 139–170.

107. N. Islam, "Pulmonary Tuberculosis in East Pakistan," *British Journal of Diseases of the Chest* 58, no. 1 (1964): 36–41.

108. G. Watts, "Wallace Fox," *The Lancet* 375, no. 9720 (2010): 1076.

109. T. McKeown, R. G. Record, and R. D. Turner, "An Interpretation of the Decline of Mortality in England and Wales during the Twentieth Century," *Population Studies* 29, no. 3 (1975): 391–422.

110. J. Colgrove, "The McKeown Thesis: A Historical Controversy and Its Enduring Influence," *American Journal of Public Health* 92, no. 5 (2002): 725–729.

111. M. Blackburn, "First Nation Infants Subject to 'Human Experimental Work' for TB Vaccine in 1930s–40s," *APTN News*, 24 July 2013.

112. D. Stuckler, L. P. King, and S. Basu, "International Monetary Fund Programs and Tuberculosis Outcomes in Post-Communist Countries," *PLoS Medicine* 5, no. 7 (2008): e143.

113. D. E. Goldberg, R. F. Siliciano, and W. R. Jacobs, "Outwitting Evolution: Fighting Drug-Resistant TB, Malaria, and HIV," *Cell* 148, no. 6 (2012): 1271–1283.

114. W. F. Paolo and J. D. Nosanchuk, "Tuberculosis in New York City: Recent Lessons and a Look Ahead," *The Lancet Infectious Diseases* 4, no. 5 (2004): 287–293.

115. T. Parish, "Steps to Address Anti-Microbial Drug Resistance in Today's Drug Discovery," *Expert Opinion on Drug Discovery* 14, no. 2 (2019): 91–94.

116. W. F. Paolo and J. D. Nosanchuk, "Tuberculosis in New York City: Recent Lessons and a Look Ahead."

117. K. J. Cummings, "Tuberculosis Control: Challenges of an Ancient and Ongoing Epidemic," *Public Health Reports* 122 (2007): 683–692.

118. M. C. Raviglione, "The TB Epidemic from 1992 to 2002," *Tuberculosis* 83, no. 1–3 (2003): 4–14.

119. D. Maher, *What Is DOTS?: A Guide to Understanding the WHO-Recommended TB Control Strategy Known as DOTS* (Geneva: World Health Organization, 1999).

120. H. T. Nguyen et al., "Strengthening Tuberculosis Control Overseas: Who Benefits?," *Value in Health* 18, no. 2 (2015): 180–188.

121. J. B. Foster et al., "Critical Consideration of Tuberculosis Management of Papua New Guinea Nationals and Cross-Border Health Issues in the Remote Torres Strait Islands, Australia," *Tropical Medicine and Infectious Disease* 7 (2022): 251.

122. I. Barberis et al., "The History of Tuberculosis: From the First Historical Records to the Isolation of Koch's Bacillus".

123. T. M. Daniel, "The History of Tuberculosis".

124. "Tuberculosis Fact Sheet," *World Health Organization*, 2021, https://www.who.int/news-room/fact-sheets/detail/tuberculosis (accessed 7 June 2022).

1 Well, That Would Be Telling...

So what's the worst disease of all time? Unsurprisingly, it stretches across history: famous deaths include the Pharaoh Tutankhamun, Dante the Italian poet, David Livingston in Zambia, the Holy Roman Emperor Henry VI, Pope Urban VII (after reigning for 13 days, the shortest papacy in history), Princess Paula of Brazil, and Oliver Cromwell. Christopher Columbus, George Washington, Abraham Lincoln, and Ulysses S. Grant all survived it.

Symptoms include acute febrile illness, chronic debilitation, complication of pregnancy, and impairment of physical development and learning in children.[1] Written references date back to China in 2700 BCE, Mesopotamian clay tablets in 200 BCE, Egyptian papyri from 1570 BCE, and Hindu texts from the sixth century BCE.[2] However, the disease is much older than that. Parasites of this disease have been found in mosquitoes preserved in amber from the Palaeogene period, approximately 30 million years ago,[3] and relatives of the disease have been found in midges (biting flies) from 100 million years ago.[4] The diversity of *Plasmodium falciparum* (the deadliest of these parasites) is greater in Africa than the rest of the world, suggesting that modern humans were suffering from it even before they left Africa.[5] Indeed, malaria has been with us throughout our entire journey as a species.

Parasites are organisms that live inside an individual and gain food from—or at the expense of—the host. In humans, malaria parasites grow and multiply first in the liver and then in the red blood cells, destroying them as they release offspring parasites. Conversely, the parasite causes no damage to the mosquito, which exchanges its infection with a host upon biting. Only the female mosquito can transmit malaria, as she uses human blood to aid in reproduction.[6] Bacteria and viruses are comparatively simple when compared to parasites. The polio virus, for example, consists of exactly 11 genes. *Plasmodium falciparum* has more than 5,000.[7]

Indeed, the disease has even affected modern-day human evolution. As a major killer of children, malaria is the strongest known force for evolutionary selection in recent history.[8] In Africa, sickle-cell trait—a gene that can cause blood disorder, leading to attacks of pain, swelling, and anaemia if it is present on both chromosomes[9]—is selected for because it protects against malaria.[10] O-type blood provides some protection against malaria, but this blood type is even older than human malaria, suggesting that it originally evolved for some reason other than malaria protection, likely in response to a now-unknown disease.[11]

There are no references to malaria in the Aztec or Mayan medical texts, suggesting that it was brought to North America by European settlers and the West Africans they enslaved.[12] It has been speculated that one of the reasons West Africans were brought to the Americas in the slave trade was because of their greater resistance to malaria. North of the Mason–Dixon line, there were fewer malaria-transmitting mosquitoes. British-indentured servants were more profitable, as they would work towards their freedom. In the South, however, the owners of large plantations came to rely on the more malaria-resistant West Africans.[13] Whereas urban conditions and industrialization gave rise to TB, malaria was and is a disease of agriculture and the rural poor.[14]

It's been a particularly persistent threat during wartime. In the Walcheren Expedition in the Netherlands, the British were conquered by malaria before a single battle could be fought.[15] Malaria caused huge losses for the British in the American South during the Revolutionary War, as well as for Union soldiers during the Civil War.[16] During the First World War, similar numbers of troops on both sides were infected, but the death rate among the Central Powers was significantly higher. Slightly more than one in every 200 infected Allied soldiers died from the disease, but more than four deaths for every hundred soldiers with malaria died among the Central Powers' troops.[17] Between 1942 and 1945, there were 492,299 cases of the disease and 302 deaths among U.S. troops, with the highest incidence of malarial attacks occurring in the India–Burma–China theatre.[18] All told, U.S. forces lost an astounding nine million man-days during that period due to the disease.[19]

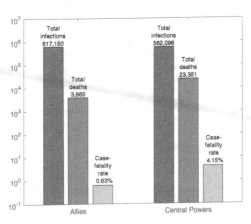

Figure 1.1. Total infections and deaths during the First World War.

Source: B. J. Brabin, 2014.[20]

The word comes from the Italian *mal'aria*, meaning "spoiled air."[21] It's spread by mosquitoes, which we now know are a vector for numerous diseases. However, this wasn't known for many centuries; for over 2,500 years, the idea persisted that malaria fevers were caused by miasmas rising from swamps.[22] Over the centuries, circumstantial evidence had accumulated that suggested that mosquitoes might be connected with malaria; by 1883, American physician Albert Freeman Africanus King had assembled a mass of evidence that came to be known as the mosquito-malaria doctrine.[23] King even proposed that a wire fence as tall as the Washington monument (then the tallest building in the world) be erected around the entire capital city. This suggestion was greeted with uproarious laughter from his colleagues, as the link between malaria and mosquitoes was not yet proven.[24]

Treatments have ranged from bloodletting,* induced vomiting, and trepanning (drilling a hole in the skull) in the Middle Ages to the use of quinine, a drug extracted from the Peruvian cinchona tree (the same ingredient that gives tonic water its bitter taste).[25] Quinine was the first chemical compound to treat an infectious disease and is considered the most serendipitous discovery of the seventeenth century.[26] South American natives chewed on the bark from the cinchona tree to stop shivering, so Jesuit priests in the 1630s guessed that it might work on malarial fevers; they got lucky, because quinine doesn't actually reduce fever, but it does cure malaria by poisoning the malaria parasite.[27] Malaria is an unusual disease in that the treatment for it was found almost 300 years before its cause and mode of transmission was discovered.[28] For 200 years, until the cinchona tree was finally established on plantations in India, Sri Lanka, and Java, the only way to acquire the cure was directly from South America.[29]

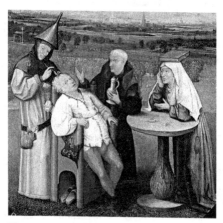

Figure 1.2. Trepanning in the Middle Ages (in this case to "cure" madness).

Source: The Extraction of the Stone of Madness by Heironymous Bosch.

After the Second World War, quinine was replaced by the drug chloroquine; subsequently, a newer and more effective set of drugs called

---

* To be fair, that treatment was applied to the majority of diseases in the Middle Ages, as seen elsewhere in this book.

artemisinins are now present in every treatment, although chloroquine is still used. Artemisinins were (re)discovered by Chinese researchers screening historical cures for fever.[30] Artemisinins were responsible for cutting African mortality in half between 2000 and 2015,[31] although it has partially rebounded.[32] Treatment with a combination of multiple anti-malarial drugs can help quell drug resistance, just as it does with HIV antiretroviral treatment (see chapter 8): if a mutant parasite resistant to one of the drugs arises during the course of infection, the parasite will be killed by the other drug in the combination.[33]

Despite the existence of multi-drug treatments for malaria, a whopping 3.3 billion people are currently at risk,[34] almost half the planet.[35] Ninety percent of deaths due to malaria occur in sub-Saharan Africa, mostly among children under five.[36] In sub-Saharan Africa, malaria costs more than one percentage point of economic growth every year.[37] Many who don't die end up scarred for life, because some strains cause cutaneous complications.[38] Other complications include scarring of the nervous system.[39] It's been suggested that, due to malaria, almost every child in Africa may be neurologically scarred in some way.[40]

So how many people have died from malaria? It's a more complicated question than it might appear. Unlike most diseases, malaria has been with us since time immemorial.[41] That gave it a lot of opportunities to kill an enormous number of humans or pre-humans. It's been speculated that malaria has killed *50 billion* humans.[42] That is an astonishing number, but what is perhaps more astonishing is that the sum total of humans—specifically *homo sapiens*—who have ever lived is around 117 billion,[43] which suggests that malaria has killed about 40% of all of us.[44] That would make it not only the worst disease of all time but the worst thing humans have ever faced.

How plausible is this? As we've seen elsewhere, most diseases are relatively new, jumping species once we started working with farm animals,[45] whereas malaria has been with us for much, much longer. So if the vast majority of humans or pre-humans died from it in all the millennia before agriculture, that might get the numbers up. On the other hand, there simply weren't that many humans at any given time back then. There were only about 18,500 humans breeding on the planet 1.2 million years ago, a period known as the population bottleneck.[46]

As you can imagine, this 50-billion estimate has been hotly debated. It was reported as early as 2002,[47] and continues to be reported,[48] though without any decisive source. Revised estimates have put the total percentage of humans killed by the disease at 4%–5%.[49] That's still around *5 billion* people, five times greater than TB. However, the high estimate might not be as outrageous as it seems. In the modern era, a malaria outbreak in the Punjab in India in 1908 killed 30%–40% of the population, as did a similar epidemic in 1892.[50]

Throughout the twentieth century, global malaria-related deaths never fell below half a million per year; they were probably at least 3 million per year during most of its first half. These figures suggest that somewhere in the region of 150–300 million people died from the effects of malaria during the previous century. With around 6 billion deaths during this period, malaria may have been a factor in 2%–5% of all deaths in the twentieth century, with up to 10% of global deaths due to malaria in the first few decades.[51] It remains endemic today, with about 400,000 deaths per year,[52] though this number has massively fallen in the past two decades. These numbers suggest the 4%–5% estimate is plausible, especially since malaria-control efforts began during this time, which reduced the overall death rate.

This is where mathematical models come in. (Don't worry, math-phobes; there are no equations here.) The great power of mathematics is that it can predict the future.[53] Aside from crystal balls, we don't really have good ways to know what's likely to happen. Modelling can make predictions, if based on data. The good news is that these data don't have to be perfect or even complete; the better the data we have, the more reliable the models. But if the data are imperfect or missing, then modelling can compensate for this, by making a range of possible predictions.[54]

If the rate of expansion can be measured and the factors that go into that expansion identified, then it's possible to determine how much those factors should be altered in order to stop the disease spreading and instead start making it shrink. For example, if we use insecticides to control mosquitoes, how often should these insecticides be applied and how strong should their effect be? By determining critical thresholds, it's possible to know how much to invest in order to achieve disease control before actually doing it, which saves resources and lives.[55]

However, the journey to widespread use of mathematical models as a tool for disease management and prediction comes via a circuitous route. Mathematical models depend on the knowledge of the biology that is used to build them, and for a long time so little was known about malaria that building even rudimentary models would not have made sense. The breakthrough was discovering that malaria was spread by mosquitoes. But when—and how—did they know that?

Charles Louis Alphonse Laveran was an unknown French army officer working in Algeria in the nineteenth century. Laveran examined the blood of 200 patients and observed crescent-shaped creatures in all cases of malaria but never in those without malaria. He also noted that quinine removed these creatures from the blood. Laveran quickly realized that he had found a parasitic protozoan, which he called *Oscillaria malariae*. He presented his findings to the French Academy of Medical Sciences in December 1880[56] but failed to persuade any of the eminent microbiologists, zoologists, or malariologists of the day that he was seeing anything other than disintegrating red blood cells. Nevertheless, by 1884 he had convinced the leading Italian malariologists that malaria was caused by a protozoan and not a bacterium.[57] Laveran was awarded the Nobel Prize for Medicine in 1907. His discovery was without precedent, as no protozoan had previously been found inhabiting any kind of human blood cell.[58]

However, the most important breakthrough came on August 20, 1897, a day still celebrated as World Mosquito Day.[59] Major Ronald Ross was a British Army officer posted to India, where he made a study of malaria. He demonstrated that a blood sucking insect could not only take up infective organisms from an infected individual but could also transmit them some time later when it fed on an uninfected host—something that was completely contrary to the received opinion of the time.[60] It took a long time before other investigators realized the universal importance of this discovery, and it was not until the first decades of the twentieth century that diseases such as African trypanosomiasis, leishmaniasis, filariasis, and loaiasis were also discovered to be transmitted by the bites of infected insects.[61] Ross won the Nobel Prize for Medicine in 1902 for this discovery.[62]

At the end of 1902, Prince Auguste d'Arenberg, president of the Suez Canal Company, asked Ross to save Ismailia, the city that was built as a base for construction of the canal. Ismailia had been gravely threatened by malaria for a long time. Ross led a sanitation drive so successful that by the following year, the city officials announced that they no longer needed mosquito nets.[63] By 1904, a whole year had passed without a single reported case of malaria in Ismailia.[64] Ross conducted similar campaigns in Greece, Mauritius, Spain, Panama, and during the First World War at various places on the battlefront.[65]

The discovery that malaria was spread by mosquitoes threw up a new challenge. It is neither possible nor desirable to eradicate all the mosquitoes. They're important for the ecosystem, so you don't want to kill them all—but even if you did want to, it would be virtually impossible to do so. One of Ross's tools was mathematical modelling.[66] His model used differential equations as an engine of change to make dynamic predictions, not just static ones directly from existing data.[67] Instead, the mechanism of interactions between variables could be used to develop a forward motion that could lead to future predictions that were not immediately obvious.

Ross used the concept of R_0, the reproduction number, to predict that malaria control did not require all the mosquitoes to be killed, only a critical number of them. If that could be done, then the disease would stop expanding and start contracting, eventually heading to zero.[68] R_0 was a concept originally developed for demographics. If two parents produced (say) 2.2 children, on average, then the population would grow, whereas if two parents only produced an average of 1.9 children, the population would be shrinking. With diseases, the threshold is 1, not 2, because it's a measure of how many individuals a single individual will infect.[69]

In 1927, biochemist William Kermack and epidemiologist Anderson McKendrick expanded Ross's model to account for stochastic effects (random fluctuations in the measurements) and calculate the final size of an epidemic.[70] The field of disease modelling has since taken off—especially once HIV appeared[71]—and has been a crucial factor in the COVID-19 response.[72]

Knowing that mosquito control could manage malaria was one thing, but how was this control actually to be achieved? Vector-borne diseases such as malaria had long been a scourge of troops worldwide, and significant efforts had been invested in various wars to develop an insecticide. Ross himself was the first to use larvicide oil in 1899 in Sierra Leone, when he sprayed kerosene on water to suffocate and poison the mosquito larvae. Another larvicide was Paris green dust, made of copper acetate and copper meta-arsenite.[73] However, such control methods were often costly and had detrimental health effects on humans and other mammals.[74]

During the Second World War, DDT (see chapter 10) was introduced in the Pacific. Unit commanders were made personally responsible for regular chemoprophylaxis of their troops, which saw malaria incidence in Papua New Guinea fall from 740 per 1,000 to just 26 per 1,000 by 1944.[75] The islands of São Tomé and Príncipe saw almost complete elimination of malaria,[76] thanks to low reproduction numbers.[77]

Due to its success, DDT was rapidly introduced into public-health and malaria-control campaigns. The entire world was sprayed with DDT for decades,[78] using a method called Indoor Residual Spraying (IRS). Since mosquitoes tend to rest nearby after feeding, they are often found inside houses, so spraying in and around dwellings is highly effective,[79] whereas direct intervention of larval breeding sites may have mixed results.[80] However, IRS cannot be used in areas devoid of structures, such as forests or swamps.[81]

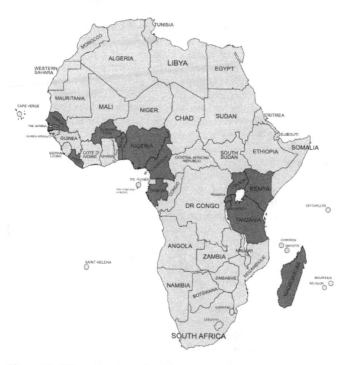

Figure 1.3. African countries with indoor residual spraying programs in the 1950s through 1970s.

Source: Created by the author using data from R. J. Smith? and S. D. Hove-Musekwa, 2008.[82]

Eradication projects in the 1950s through the 1970s in a variety of African countries demonstrated that malaria was highly responsive to control by IRS. The application of IRS consistently over time in large areas altered the vector distribution and subsequently the epidemiological pattern of malaria in Botswana, Namibia, South Africa, Swaziland, and Zimbabwe.[83] IRS resulted in the suppression of *Anopheles funestus* in some areas of the continent, removing it as a vector for transmission of malaria.[84] It was the intervention of choice in areas of particular economic interest that require a rapid and effective prevention, where financial and logistic constraints do not prevail, such as tourism, mining, oil extraction, and agricultural schemes.[85] As a result of all this spraying, malaria was eradicated from the United States by 1951 and Europe declared malaria-free in 1975.[86] However, DDT was not just used for malaria control; it was also used for agricultural purposes to control a variety of insects, with large quantities of it being dropped from crop-dusting planes.[87]

As mentioned in chapter 3, malaria was one of four diseases targeted for eradication in the twentieth century. Despite being cost-beneficial and having broad societal and political support, malaria-eradication efforts failed due to a combination of factors, including insecticide resistance, economic under development, non-human primate reservoirs, and the discontinuation of DDT as a method of vector control, following publication of Rachel Carson's *Silent Spring*.[88]

Silent Spring was the book that launched the environmental movement.[89] It strongly criticized the overuse of DDT in agriculture, noting for example that eagles' eggs were now too thin to allow eaglets to survive. However, the book only mentions malaria once, in passing.[90] DDT was banned for agricultural use in 1972; its discontinuation was a major factor in the comeback of the bald eagle and the peregrine falcon from near extinction in the U.S.[91] DDT was never banned for malaria use and poses no known ecological dangers when sprayed for malaria,[92] but it became nearly impossible to procure. It's been estimated that the ban on DDT may have killed 20 million children.[93]

The reliance on a single technological solution to malaria came at the cost of ignoring the sociopolitical context of the disease. Malaria disappeared from 39% of the targeted countries, never to return in many cases.[94] However, the uneven patterns of eradication had further effects: control of the disease became synonymous with control of communism and the spread of democracy,[95] with previously landless peasants becoming successful farmers on the newly reclaimed land. Biomedicine became the key to progress in the modern world.[96]

Other insecticides have since been used, but mosquitoes have developed resistance to them, along with DDT. Malaria was all but eliminated in Sri Lanka in the 1950s, thanks to DDT, but by the end of the 1960s, resistance to the chemical resulted in half a million cases per year.[97] Resistance is essentially an arms race: can we produce new insecticides faster than mosquitoes can evolve around them? Furthermore, the use of insecticides often has a disproportionate suppression effect on insect predators, allowing mosquitoes an evolutionary advantage.[98] Despite resistance, spraying with multiple insecticides has been successful in controlling mosquito species *Anopheles funestus*, *Anopheles gambiae*, and *Anopheles melas* in Equatorial Guinea, for example.[99]

A newer problem is global warming. Mosquitoes breed and bite more rapidly the warmer it is.[100] This means that we need to spray ever more frequently just to stand still.[101] Geographic patterns of spread also change with global warming;[102] malaria was eradicated in Australia by 1981[103] but re-entered the far northern parts in 1996 and 2002, as mosquito habitats shifted.[104]

Other solutions have been attempted. A low-tech solution involves polystyrene bean bag balls floating in liquid waste in open toilets, which stops the mosquitoes from breeding but allows solid waste to pass through.[105] Another one is to simply sleep beneath a bednet, since most mosquitoes bite at night. Bednets are not a new idea; the Egyptian Pharaoh Sneferu (who reigned from 2613–2589 BCE) used bednets as protection, as did Cleopatra VII, the last pharaoh (69–30 BCE, ruled 51–30 BCE).[106]

A recent breakthrough has been a combination of the two: insecticide-treated bednets mix a physical barrier with a chemical one. They've been especially good at reducing child mortality and have been responsible for a massive reduction in malaria cases in the past 20 years.[107] Naturally, there are always quirks. Insecticide-treated bednets have been provided for free to many villages, but these are not always used as intended; people have used the nets for fishing,[108] for example, which illustrates the complexity of attempting to solve one issue (malaria) without thinking through its interaction with others (hunger).

A proposed idea has been to breed genetically modified mosquitoes that can interbreed with regular mosquitoes, but which die before the malaria parasite can develop inside them. It takes 10–12 days for the parasite to develop within a mosquito and reach the salivary glands. This genetic manipulation causes cells in the mosquito gut to secrete proteins that delay parasite development.[109] Such approaches have already been implemented in Brazil, Panama, Malaysia, and the United States for mosquitoes that carry dengue, Zika, and yellow fever.[110] This was not the first attempt at biological control of malaria: in the first half of the twentieth century, mosquitofish (so named for its predilection for eating mosquito larvae) were brought from North America to regions all around the world, including South America, Palestine, Italy, and Central Asia, in an attempt to control mosquito populations.[111] Another genetic modification is to make all female offspring infertile, so that the mosquito population could be wiped out. While the first option has not been implemented in the wild for malaria-specific mosquitoes, the latter has seen millions of genetically modified male mosquitoes released in Brazil.[112]

Sadly, when COVID-19 interrupted supply chains of health commodities, malaria-control efforts were severely curtailed,[113] which could lead to an explosion in malaria deaths.[114] The same thing had previously happened in 2014 when the Ebola epidemic disrupted the distribution of insecticide-treated bednets.[115] It's a good illustration of how disease-control efforts intersect and overlap, as well as a reminder that each disease does not exist in isolation.

However, there's new hope on the horizon. The RTS,S malaria vaccine—developed in the late 1980s at SmithKline Biologicals in Belgium, later developed by GlaxoSmithKline and the Walter Reed Army Institute of Research in the United States, with clinical trials that began in 2012—is currently being rolled out throughout Africa, having started in 2019.[116] It's the first parasitic vaccine ever developed,[117] which is something of a modern-day miracle, given the complexity of parasitic infection.[118] The major issue with the vaccine at the moment is cost: at five dollars a dose, it's a bargain compared to most vaccines, but still vastly more expensive than most people who need it can afford.[119]

This vaccine is what's called a disease-modifying vaccine: it (usually) allows you to become infected, but it makes the progression of the disease less bad when you do get it. You're less sick when you catch it, less likely to die, and recover faster. What's particularly helpful about such a vaccine for malaria is that the disease primarily kills children under five, so holding back death for a few years can make an enormous difference. These kinds of vaccines aren't perfect, but they're incredibly valuable. It's thought that the most likely HIV vaccine, if one appears, will also be a disease-modifying vaccine.[120]

Whether it's killed 5 billion or 50 billion, malaria is one of the worst things we've ever faced as a species. However, it's much less of a threat today and almost non-existent in developed countries. We have mathematical modelling and DDT to thank for that. Someday, hopefully, we'll be able to add vaccination to that list.

Notes

1. J. Keiser et al., "Urbanization in sub-Saharan Africa and Implication for Malaria Control," *American Journal of Tropical Medicine & Hygiene* 7, suppl. 2 (2004): 118–127.
2. F. E. Cox, "History of the Discovery of the Malaria Parasites and their Vectors," *Parasites & Vectors* 3, no. 1 (2010): 1–9.
3. G. Poinar, "*Plasmodium dominicana* n. sp. (Plasmodiidae: Haemospororida) from Tertiary Dominican Amber," *Systematic Parasitology* 61, no. 1 (2005): 47–52.
4. M. Wayne and B. Bolker, *Infectious Diseases: A Very Short Introduction* (Oxford: Oxford University Press, 2015).
5. T. Higham, *The World before Us: How Science Is Revealing a New Story of Our Human Origins* (London: Penguin, 2021).
6. F. E. Cox, "History of the Discovery of the Malaria Parasites and Their Vectors".
7. M. Finkel, "Malaria: Stopping a Global Killer," *National Geographic*, July 2007.
8. D. P. Kwiatkowski, "How Malaria Has Affected the Human Genome and What Human Genetics Can Teach Us about Malaria," *American Journal of Human Genetics* 77, no. 2 (2006): 171–192.
9. M. J. Stuart and R. L. Nagel, "Sickle-Cell Disease," *The Lancet* 364, no. 9442 (2004): 1343–1360.
10. D. P. Kwiatkowski, "How Malaria Has Affected the Human Genome and What Human Genetics Can Teach Us about Malaria".
11. M. Wayne and B. Bolker, *Infectious Diseases*.
12. F. E. Cox, "History of the Discovery of the Malaria Parasites and Their Vectors".
13. G. Bertocchi and A. Dimico, "Slavery, Education, and Inequality," *European Economic Review* 70 (2014): 197–209.
14. C. W. McMillen, *Pandemics: A Very Short Introduction* (Oxford: Oxford University Press, 2016).
15. M. R. Howard, "Walcheren 1809: A Medical Catastrophe," *British Medical Journal* 319, no. 7225 (1999): 1642–1645.
16. V. J. Cirillo, "Two Faces of Death: Fatalities from Disease and Combat in America's Principal Wars, 1775 to Present," *Perspectives in Biology and Medicine* 51, no. 1 (2008): 121–133.
17. B. J. Brabin, "Malaria's Contribution to World War One—The Unexpected Adversary," *Malaria Journal* 13 (2014): 497.
18. V. J. Cirillo, "Two Faces of Death: Fatalities from Disease and Combat in America's Principal Wars, 1775 to Present".
19. L. J. Bruce-Chwatt, "Mosquitoes, Malaria and War: Then and Now," *Journal of the Royal Army Medical Corps* 131 (1985): 85–99.
20. B. J. Brabin, "Malaria's Contribution to World War One—The Unexpected Adversary," *Malaria Journal* 13 (2014): 497.
21. F. E. Cox, "History of the Discovery of the Malaria Parasites and Their Vectors".
22. M. Finkel, "Malaria: Stopping a Global Killer".

23. A. F. A. King, "Insects and Disease: Mosquitoes and Malaria," *Popular Science Monthly* 23 (1883): 644–658.

24. S. T. Charles, "Albert FA King (1841–1914), an Armchair Scientist," *Journal of the History of Medicine and Allied Sciences* 24, no. 1 (1969): 22–36.

25. D. Bhattacharjee and G. Shivaprakash, "Drug Resistance in Malaria—In a Nutshell," *Journal of Applied Pharmaceutical Science* 6, no. 3 (2016): 137–143.

26. J. Achan et al., "Quinine, an Old Anti-Malarial Drug in a Modern World: Role in the Treatment of Malaria," *Malaria Journal* 10 (2011): 144.

27. M. Wayne and B. Bolker, *Infectious Diseases.*

28. N. Harrison, "In Celebration of the Jesuit's Powder: A History of Malaria Treatment," *The Lancet Infectious Diseases* 15, no. 10 (2015): 1143.

29. M. Finkel, "Malaria: Stopping a Global Killer".

30. M. Wayne and B. Bolker, *Infectious Diseases.*

31. P. W. Gething et al., "Mapping *Plasmodium falciparum* Mortality in Africa between 1990 and 2015," *New England Journal of Medicine* 375 (2016): 2435–2445.

32. P. J. Rosenthal, "Are Artemisinin-Based Combination Therapies for Malaria Beginning to Fail in Africa?," *The American Journal of Tropical Medicine and Hygiene* 105, no. 4 (2021): 857–858.

33. G. Kokwaro, "Ongoing Challenges in the Management of Malaria," *Malaria Journal* 8, suppl. 1 (2009): S2.

34. K. E. Battle and J. K. Baird, "The Global Burden of *Plasmodium vivax* Malaria Is Obscure and Insidious," *PLoS Medicine* 18, no. 10 (2021): e1003799.

35. A. D. Lopez et al., "Global and Regional Burden of Disease and Risk Factors, 2001: Systematic Analysis of Population Health Data," *The Lancet* 367, no. 9524 (2006): 1747–1757.

36. P. van de Perre and J.-P. Dedet, "Vaccine Efficacy: Winning a Battle (Not War) against Malaria," *The Lancet* 364, no. 9443 (2004): 1411–1420.

37. J. Keiser et al., "Urbanization in Sub-Saharan Africa and Implication for Malaria Control".

38. A. Chaudhary et al., "Cutaneous Manifestations of Malaria," *BMJ Case Reports* 15, no. 6 (2022): e251257.

39. M. H. Deininger et al., "Accumulation of Endostatin/CollagenXVIII in Brains of Patients Who Died with Cerebral Malaria," *Journal of Neuroimmunology* 131 (2002): 216–221.

40. M. Finkel, "Malaria: Stopping a Global Killer".

41. G. Poinar, "*Plasmodium dominicana* n. sp. (Plasmodiidae: Haemospororida) from Tertiary Dominican Amber," *Systematic Parasitology* 61, no. 1 (2005): 47–52.

42. M. Finkel, "Malaria: Stopping a Global Killer".

43. T. Kaneda and C. Haub, "How Many People Have Ever Lived on Earth?," *The Pledge for Racial and Ethnic Equality*, 18 May 2021.

44. S. Callahan, "Forget Sharks—Mosquitoes Are the Deadliest Maneaters on Earth," *New York Post*, 3 August 2019.

45. B. A. Jones et al., "Zoonosis Emergence Linked to Agricultural Intensification and Environmental Change," *Proceedings of the National Academy of Sciences* 110, no. 21 (2013): 8399–8404.

46. A. Gibbons, "Human Ancestors Were an Endangered Species," *Science*, 19 January 2010.

47. J. Whitfield, "Portrait of a Serial Killer," *Nature*, 3 October 2002.

48. B. Bethune, "The Mosquito Has Killed Billions and Changed Our DNA—And It's Going to Get Worse," *Macleans*, 10 July 2019.

49. R. Pomeroy, "Has Malaria really Killed Half of Everyone Who Ever Lived?," *Real Clear Science*, 3 October 2019.

50. S. R. Christophers, "What Disease Costs India: Being a Statement of the Problem before Medical Research in India," *The Indian Medical Gazette* 59 (1924): 196–200.

51. R. Carter and K. M. Mendis, "Evolutionary and Historical Aspects of the Burden of Malaria," *Clinical Microbiology Reviews* 15, no. 4 (2002): 564–594.

52. *World Malaria Report 2020: 20 Years of Global Progress and Challenges* (Geneva: World Health Organization, 2020).

53. R. J. Smith?, "What Can Zombies Teach Us about Mathematics?," *The Partner* 47 (2012).

54. F. Brauer, "Mathematical Epidemiology Is Not an Oxymoron," *BMC Public Health* 9 (2009): S2.

55. R. J. Smith? and S. D. Hove-Musekwa, "Determining Effective Spraying periods to Control Malaria via Indoor Residual Spraying in Sub-Saharan Africa," *Journal of Applied Mathematics and Decision Sciences* 2008 (2008): 745463.

56. A. Laveran, "Un nouveau parasite trouvé dans le sang de malades atteints de fièvre palustre. Origine parasitaire des accidents de l'impaludisme," *Bulletins et Mémoires de la Société Médicale des Hôpitaux de Paris* 17 (1881): 158–164.

57. A. Laveran, *Traité des Fiévres Palustres avec la Description des Microbes du Paludisme* (Paris: Doin, 1884).

58. F. E. Cox, "History of the Discovery of the Malaria Parasites and Their Vectors".

59. C. Fornandel, "World Mosquito Day 2021—20th August 2021," *IVCC*, 18 August 2021.

60. E. Nye and M. Gibson, *Ronald Ross: Malariologist and Polymath: A Biography* (Houndmills: MacMillan, 1997).

61. F. E. Cox, "History of the Discovery of the Malaria Parasites and Their Vectors".

62. E. Nye and M. Gibson, *Ronald Ross*.

63. R. Ross and R. Boyce, "The Antimalaria Campaign at Ismailia," *British Medical Journal* 1, no. 2256 (1904): 760.

64. R. Ross, "Malaria in Cyprus and Greece," *Proceedings of the Royal Society of Medicine* 7, no. 5 (1914): 107–118.

65. E. Bendiner, "Ronald Ross and the Mystery of Malaria," *Hospital Practice* 29, no. 10 (1994): 95–112.

66. S. Mandal, R. R. Sarkar, and S. Sinha, "Mathematical Models of Malaria—A Review," *Malaria Journal* 10 (2011): 202.

67. N. Bacaër, *A Short History of Mathematical Population Dynamics* (London: Springer, 1911).

68. R. Ross, *Studies on Malaria* (London: John Murray, 1928).

69. J. A. Heesterbeek, "A Brief History of R_0 and a Recipe for Its Calculation," *Acta Biotheoretica* 50, no. 3 (2002): 189–204.

70. N. Bacaër, *A Short History of Mathematical Population Dynamics*.

71. L. F. Johnson and P. J. White, "A Review of Mathematical Models of HIV/AIDS Interventions and Their Implications for Policy," *Sexually Transmitted Infections* 87, no. 7 (2011): 629–634.

72. E. S. McBryde et al., "Role of Modelling in COVID-19 Policy Development," *Paediatric Respiratory Reviews* 35 (2020): 57–60.

73. G. Majori, "The Long Road to Malaria Eradication," *The Lancet* 354 (1999): SIV31.

74. F. S. Lisella, K. R. Long, and H. G. Scott, "Health Aspects of Arsenicals in the Environment," *Journal of Environmental Health* 34, no. 5 (1972): 511–518.

75. L. J. Bruce-Chwatt, "Mosquitoes, Malaria and War: Then and Now," *Journal of the Royal Army Medical Corps* 131 (1985): 85–99.

76. H. D. Teklehaimanot et al., "Malaria in Sao Tome and Principe: On the Brink of Elimination after Three Years of Effective Antimalarial Measures," *The American Journal of Tropical Medicine and Hygiene* 80, no. 1 (2009): 133–140.

77. R. Hagmann et al., "Malaria and Its Possible Control on the Island of Príncipe," *Malaria Journal* 2 (2003): 15.

78. P. I. Trigg and A. V. Kondrachine, "Malaria Control in the 1990s," *Bulletin of the World Health Organization* 76 (1998): 11–16.

79. K. Macintyre et al., "Rolling Out Insecticide Treated Nets in Eritrea: Examining the Determinants of Possession and Use in Malarious Zones during the Rainy Season," *Tropical Medicine and International Health* 11, no. 6 (2006): 824–833.

80. U. Fillinger et al., "Integrated Malaria Vector Control with Microbial Larvicides and Insecticide-Treated Nets in Western Kenya: A Controlled Trial," *Bulletin of the World Health Organization* 87 (2009): 655–665.

81. M. Al-arydah and R. J. Smith?, "Controlling Malaria with Indoor Residual Spraying in Spatially Heterogeneous Environments," *Mathematical Biosciences and Engineering* 8, no. 4 (2011): 889–914.

82. R. J. Smith? and S. D. Hove-Musekwa, "Determining Effective Spraying Periods to Control Malaria via Indoor Residual Spraying in Sub-Saharan Africa".

83. R. L. Kouznetsov, "Malaria Control by Application of Indoor Spraying of Residual Insecticides in Tropical Africa and Its Impact on Population Health," *Tropical Doctor* 7, no. 2 (1977): 81–91.

84. B. Abong'o et al., "Impact of Indoor Residual Spraying with Pirimiphos-Methyl (Actellic 300CS) on Entomological Indicators of Transmission and Malaria Case Burden in Migori County, Western Kenya," *Scientific Reports* 10 (2020): 4518.

85. "Indoor Residual Spraying: An Operational Manual for Indoor Residual Spraying (IRS) for Malaria Transmission Control and Elimination," *World Health Organization*, 2015.

86. K. Migiro, "Timeline: The Long Road to Malaria Eradication," *Reuters*, 8 June 2016.

87. G. F. Burnett, C. W. Lee, and P. O. Park, "Aircraft Applications of Insecticides in East Africa. XV.—Very-Low-Volume Treatment of a Seed-Bean Crop with DDT in Oil Solution," *Bulletin of Entomological Research* 56, no. 4 (1966): 701–714.

88. B. Aylward et al., "When Is a Disease Eradicable? 100 Years of Lessons Learned," *American Journal of Public Health* 90, no. 10 (2000): 1515–1520.

89. C. S. Berry-Cabán, "DDT and Silent Spring: Fifty Years After," *Journal of Military and Veterans' Health* 19, no. 4 (is there a year?): 19–24.

90. R. Carson, *Silent Spring* (Boston: Houghton Mifflin, 1962).

91. R. Tren and R. Bate, *When Politics Kills: Malaria and the DDT Story* (Washington, DC: Competitive Enterprise Institute, 2001).

92. J. D. Sachs, "A New Global Effort to Control Malaria," *Science* 298, no. 5591 (2002): 122–124.

93. M. Finkel, "Malaria: Stopping a Global Killer".

94. C. W. McMillen, *Pandemics*.

95. R. M. Packard, "Malaria Dreams: Postwar Visions of Health and Development in the Third World," *Medical Anthropology* 17, no. 3 (1997): 279–296.

96. C. W. McMillen, *Pandemics*.

97. K. Kupferschmidt, "After 40 Years, the Most Important Weapon against Mosquitoes May Be Failing," *Science News*, 13 October 2016.

98. L. J. Bruce-Chwatt, "Mosquitoes, Malaria and War: Then and Now".

99. B. L. Sharp et al., "Malaria Vector Control by Indoor Residual Insecticide Spraying on the Tropical Island of Bioko, Equatorial Guinea," *Malaria Journal* 6 (2007): 52.

100. B. Wudel and E. Shadabi, "A Short Review of Literature on the Effects of Climate Change on Mosquito-Borne Illnesses in Canada," *National Collaborating Centre for Infectious Diseases* 278 (2016): 1–10.

101. R. J. Smith? and S. D. Hove-Musekwa, "Determining Effective Spraying Periods to Control Malaria via Indoor Residual Spraying in Sub-Saharan Africa".

102. B. Wudel and E. Shadabi, "A Short Review of Literature on the Effects of Climate Change on Mosquito-Borne Illnesses in Canada".

103. J. H. Bryan, D. H. Foley, and R. W. Sutherst, "Malaria Transmission and Climate Change in Australia," *Medical Journal of Australia* 164, no. 6 (1996): 345–347.

104. Queensland Health, *Queensland Health Guidelines for Public Health Units: Malaria*, September 2011, https://www.health.qld.gov.au/cdcg/index/malaria (accessed 21 June 2022)

105. N. Sivagnaname, D. D. Amalraj, and T. Mariappan, "Utility of Expanded Polystyrene (EPS) Beads in the Control of Vector-Borne Diseases," *Indian Journal of Medical Research* 122, no. 4 (2005): 291–296.

106. D. Rawal, "An Overview of Natural History of the Human Malaria," *International Journal of Mosquito Research* 7, no. 2 (2020): 8–10.

107. J. Pryce, M. Richardson, and C. Lengeler, "Insecticide-Treated Nets for Preventing Malaria," *Cochrane Database of Systematic Reviews* 11 (2018): CD0003.

108. G. Kokwaro, "Ongoing Challenges in the Management of Malaria," *Malaria Journal* 8 (2009): S2.

109. M. Le Page, "Mosquitoes Are Being Genetically Modified so They Can't Spread Malaria," *New Scientist*, 21 September 2022.

110. E. Waltz, "First Genetically Modified Mosquitoes Released in the United States," *Nature* 593 (2021): 175–176.

111. M. Wayne and B. Bolker, *Infectious Diseases*.

112. M. Le Page, "Mosquitoes Are Being Genetically Modified so They Can't Spread Malaria".

113. A. T. Aborode et al., "Fighting COVID-19 at the Expense of Malaria in Africa: The Consequences and Policy Options," *The American Journal of Tropical Medicine and Hygiene* 104, no. 1 (2021): 26–29.

114. O. Dyer, "African Malaria Deaths Set to Dwarf COVID-19 Fatalities as Pandemic Hits Control Efforts, WHO Warns," *British Medical Journal* 371 (2020): m4711.

115. P. G. Walker, M. T. White, and J. T. Griffin, "Malaria Morbidity and Mortality in Ebola-Affected Countries Caused by Decreased Health-Care Capacity, and the Potential Effect of Mitigation Strategies: A Modelling Analysis," *The Lancet Infectious Diseases* 15 (2015): 825–832.

116. M. B. Laurens, "RTS, S/AS01 Vaccine (Mosquirix™): An Overview," *Human Vaccines & Immunotherapeutics* 16, no. 3 (2020): 480–489.

117. G. Vogel, "WHO Gives First Malaria Vaccine the Green Light," *Science* 374, no. 6565 (2021): 245–246.

118. D. L. Doolan and S. L. Hoffman, "The Complexity of Protective Immunity against Liver-Stage Malaria," *The Journal of Immunology* 165, no. 3 (2000): 1453–1462.

119. G. Vogel, "WHO Gives First Malaria Vaccine the Green Light".

120. R. J. Smith? and S. M. Blower, "Could Disease-Modifying HIV Vaccines Cause Population-Level Perversity?," *The Lancet Infectious Diseases* 4, no. 10 (2004): 636–639.

Lessons Learned
and the Way Forward

In 1963, in the wake of DDT, antibiotics, and vaccination campaigns, T. Aidan Cockburn, an infectious disease specialist, claimed "We can look forward with confidence to a considerable degree of freedom from infectious diseases at a time not too far in the future. Indeed, it seems reasonable to anticipate that within some measurable time [...] all the major infections will have disappeared."[1] Sadly, his words seem overly optimistic today.

As the chapters in this book collectively illustrate, infectious diseases have been a constant scourge to humanity throughout history. They've wreaked havoc in terms of enormous death tolls, which we've tracked, but also massive amounts of suffering and disability. They've been present throughout history and in every part of the world, shaping and reshaping societies and culture throughout human existence.

However, as also illustrated throughout this book, innovative solutions—many of them low-tech—combining scientific insight with cultural sensitivity, are what allow us to make progress. Combinations of new technology, innovative thinking, behaviour changes, and vaccinations have turned the tide on many of these diseases, leading to vastly expanded life expectancies and quality of life for many people in various parts of the world. Vaccines have been a crucial tool in fighting diseases, but they aren't the only one, nor is the invention of a vaccine sufficient. Public engagement is also crucial, in order to dispel fears of new technologies. Older ideas for eradication involving education, case management, and vector control have proven their worth in more recent times as well. The future will likely require a mix of old and new ideas, working hand in hand.

Breakthroughs in identifying the causative agents of TB, plague, or malaria happened many hundreds or thousands of years after the diseases had started circulating. Compare that to the biomedical triumph of identifying HIV as the cause of AIDS a mere two years after its discovery, illustrating the payoff from decades of advances in immunology, molecular biology, and virology.

Disease control is often a case of two steps forward, one step back. While advances in technology are welcome, backlash borne of ignorance and misinformation can do irreparable damage to the cause. Existing societal inequalities such as racism, misogyny, and class barriers both propagate disease and are exacerbated by its existence. There's no silver bullet that stops a pandemic in its tracks. Instead, we make progress when we apply a variety of techniques, each chipping away at some aspect until the problem can be wrestled into submission.

The arrival of COVID-19 taught us that, despite our technological advancements, we are highly susceptible to new infections that can be transmitted around the globe. Modern infrastructure allows infectious diseases to travel at unprecedented speeds. Social media allow conspiracy theories and unchecked misinformation to travel even faster. These are the new enemies in an ancient fight that humanity has waged since time immemorial; sometimes successfully, often not.

How can we stave off future pandemics? They may be unavoidable, but, as the examples of the 1976 swine flu outbreak, the 2003 monkeypox cases, and the 2003 SARS epidemic illustrate, it's possible to stop a pandemic before it starts. This requires vigilance, swift action, mobilizing governments, public engagement, and a healthy dose of luck.

Future challenges include climate change, factory farming, risky research, artificial intelligence, and others that are beyond our current ability to grasp. How these will facilitate the rise of new outbreaks or new mutations of existing diseases remains to be seen. Diseases are remarkably adaptable, so they will doubtless march in lockstep with our changing society, just as we will attempt to fight them through ever-more-innovative methods.

Advances in living standards, food abundance, water quality, and infant survival have had the incidental effect of substantially combatting infectious diseases. While such improvements may not be specifically geared towards fighting pandemics, improvements at the lowest levels of society benefit everyone. You may have noticed that many chapters mention famous names who were killed by the disease in question; the exceptions are chapters 9 and 10, because I could find not a single individual from the Third Plague or cocoliztli whose name we know. That's largely because these diseases primarily affected the poor, the disenfranchised, and non-Western societies. That in itself is its own tragedy, beyond the sheer awfulness of the body count.

This book has been titled *The Top Ten Diseases of All Time*, partly because infectious diseases are fascinating unto themselves, partly because there was no accurate record of the sheer numbers killed, and partly because it gives the book a structure. However, it's important to note that these are not just numbers but people. Human beings, with hopes and dreams and fears, cut short before their time because of epidemics and pandemics, only some of which we've conquered. Hopefully, the engaging title is nevertheless a gateway to a) remembering that those people lived and died and b) hoping that we can learn to avoid the fates that befell them.

On a broader scale, infectious diseases have reshaped societies, both directly and indirectly. Creative solutions to pandemics have resulted in technological developments, art, music, philosophy, and daily practices that have become embedded in our culture. Some of these have been unambiguously positive; others are more complicated. We can only hope that such progress continues as we meet more challenges. Infectious diseases will always be with us, but so is our ability to face them.

Notes

1.   T.A. Cockburn, *The Evolution and Eradication of Infectious Diseases* (Baltimore: Johns Hopkins University Press, 1963).

Further Reading

Baker, G. P. *Justinian: The Last Roman Emperor*. Lanham: Cooper Square Press, 2002.

Barnes, D. S. *The Making of a Social Disease: Tuberculosis in Nineteenth-Century France*. Berkeley: University of California Press, 1995.

Benedict, C. *Bubonic Plague in Eighteenth-Century China*. Stanford: Stanford University Press, 1996.

Busvine, J. *Disease Transmission by Insects: Its Discovery and 90 Years of Effort to Prevent It*. New York: Springer, 2012.

Crosby, A. W. *America's Forgotten Pandemic: The Influenza of 1918*. Cambridge: Cambridge University Press, 2003.

Evans, J. A. S. *The Age of Justinian: The Circumstances of Imperial Power*. New York: Routledge, 1996.

Frank, R. *The Forgotten Plague: How the Battle against Tuberculosis Was Won—And Lost*. Boston: Little, Brown and Company, 1993.

Hopkins, D. R. *The Greatest Killer: Smallpox in History*. Chicago: University of Chicago Press, 2002.

Koplow, D. A. *Smallpox: The Fight to Eradicate a Global Scourge*. Berkeley: University of California Press, 2003.

Loddenkemper, R., and J. F. Murray. *Tuberculosis and War: Lessons Learned from World War II*. Basel: Karger, 2018.

McMillen, C. W. *Pandemics: A Very Short Introduction*. Oxford: Oxford University Press, 2016.

Nye, E., and M. Gibson. *Ronald Ross: Malariologist and Polymath: A Biography*. Houndmills: MacMillan, 1997.

Orent, W. *Plague: The Mysterious Past and Mystifying Future of the World's Most Dangerous Disease*. New York: Free Press, 2004.

Pepin, J. *The Origins of AIDS*. Cambridge: Cambridge University Press, 2021.

Rajagopalan, A. H. *Portraying the Aztec Past: The Codices Boturini, Azcatitlan, and Aubin*. Austin: University of Texas Press, 2018.

Ross, R. *Studies on Malaria*. London: John Murray, 1928.

Scheidel W. *The Great Leveler*. Princeton: Princeton University Press, 2017.

Starling, A., F. Ho, L. Luke, S. Tso, and E. Yu. *Plague, SARS and the Story of Medicine in Hong Kong*. Hong Kong: Hong Kong University Press, 2006.

Taylor, M. W. *Viruses and Man: A History of Interactions*. Cham: Springer, 2014.

Throp, C. *The Horrors of the Bubonic Plague*. North Mankato: Capstone Press, 2017.

Treichler, P. A. *How to Have Theory in an Epidemic: Cultural Chronicles of AIDS*. Durham: Duke University Press, 1999.

Twigg, G. *The Black Death: A Biological Reappraisal*. New York: Schocken Books, 1985.

Wayne, M., and B. Bolker. *Infectious Diseases: A Very Short Introduction* Oxford: Oxford University Press, 2015.

Index

About the Author

Stacey Smith? (the question mark is part of her name) is a professor of disease modelling at the University of Ottawa. Using mathematics, she studies infectious diseases such as HIV, malaria, human papillomavirus, COVID-19, influenza, neglected tropical diseases—and zombies. She has published over 130 academic articles; is a winner of a Guinness World Record for her work on modelling a zombie invasion; was the winner of the 2015 Mathematics Ambassador Award, given by Canada's Partners in Research Association; won the 2018 Society for Mathematical Biology Distinguished Service Award for exceptional contribution to the field of mathematical biology and its advancement outside of research; and was awarded a 2021 prize for her outstanding contributions to the advancement of diversity, equity, inclusion, and justice at the Society for Mathematical Biology Annual Meeting. She was the first University of Ottawa employee to transition—but won't be the last! She has more than 20 books to her name, including several guides to the wonderful world of *Doctor Who: Bookwyrm* (ATB Publishing); *Who Is the Doctor*, *Who's 50*, and *The Doctors Are In* (ECW Press); *Look at the Size of That Thing!* (Pencil Tip Publishing); as well as a Black Archive on *Doctor Who and the Silurians* (Obverse Books). She's also the editor extraordinaire of the *Outside In* series of pop-culture reviews with a twist (ATB Publishing), covering *Doctor Who*, *Star Trek*, *Buffy*, *Angel*, *Firefly*, *Twin Peaks*, and *The X-Files*. Oh, and she's the world's leading expert on the transmission of Bieber Fever, but let's not worry about that one.

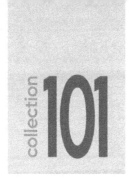

Series editor: Stacey Smith?

Join us for this new series matching academic rigour with accessibility. Featuring topics that speak to the general public but written by experts in the field in an engaging and lively style, *Collection 101* is a new vision of what academic writing can be—and who it can appeal to. Each book showcases a topic of broad interest, written simultaneously for the enthusiastic novice and the serious expert, but is designed to reach further and aim higher than most academic texts.

Recent titles in the *Collection 101* Series

Dianne Conrad, *Seniors' Learning in the Digital Age*, 2022.

Heather N. Nicol and Andrew Chater, eds., *North America's Arctic Borders: A World of Change?*, 2021.

Geoffrey Hale and Greg Anderson, eds., *Canada's Fluid Borders: Trade, Investment, Travel Migration*, 2021.

Claire-Jehanne Dubouloz Wilner, *Transformative Physical Rehabilitation*, 2020.

Zijad Delic, *Islam in the West: Beyond Integration*, 2018.

For a complete list of University of Ottawa Press titles, visit
www.press.uOttawa.ca